Copyright © 2020 by Candace Lavergne - All rights reserved.

The content contained within this book may not be reproduced, duplicated, or transmitted without direct written permission from the author or the publisher.

Under no circumstances will any blame or legal responsibility be held against the publisher, or author, for any damages, reparation, or monetary loss due to the information contained within this book, either directly or indirectly.

Legal Notice:

This book is copyright protected. It is only for personal use. You cannot amend, distribute, sell, use, quote or paraphrase any part, or the content within this book, without the consent of the author or publisher.

Disclaimer Notice:

Please note the information contained within this document is for educational and entertainment purposes only. All effort has been executed to present accurate, up to date, reliable, complete information. No warranties of any kind are declared or implied. Readers acknowledge that the author is not engaged in the rendering of legal, financial, medical, or professional advice. The content within this book has been derived from various sources. Please consult a licensed professional before attempting any techniques outlined in this book.

By reading this document, the reader agrees that under no circumstances is the author responsible for any losses, direct or indirect, that are incurred as a result of the use of the information contained within this document, including, but not limited to, errors, omissions, or inaccuracies.

CONTENTS

- Introduction 7
- The Benefits of The Instant Pot 7
- How to Use the Instant Pot? 8
- Instant Pot FAQs 9
- Mouthwatering Breakfast Recipes 10
  - Sweet Potato Hash 10
  - Bacon Ranch Potatoes 10
  - Saucy Spanish Chorizo and Potato Hash 10
  - Loaded Breakfast Potatoes 10
  - Cheesy Egg Bake 11
  - Lemon Blueberry Breakfast Cake 11
  - Bacon and Cheese Crustless Quiche 11
  - Eggs Benedict Casserole 11
  - Instant Pot Huevos Rancheros 12
  - Mexican-Style Quiche 12
  - Easy Irish Oatmeal 12
  - Spinach and Ham Frittata 12
  - Eggs En Cocotte 13
  - 5-Ingredient Cheesy Egg Bake 13
  - Instant Pot Slow Cooker Chocolate Oatmeal ... 13
  - Breakfast Espresso Oatmeal 13
  - Fruited Steel-Cut Breakfast Oats 13
  - Trail Mix Breakfast Oatmeal 14
  - Simple Breakfast Oatmeal with Brown Sugar .. 14
  - Ham and Cheese Casserole 14
  - Western Omelet Quiche 14
  - French Baked Eggs 14
  - Poached Eggs in Bell Pepper Cups 15
  - Mexican Egg Casserole 15
  - Sausage and Egg Breakfast Casserole Burritos 15
  - Yogurt with Fruits 16
  - Vanilla Apple Cinnamon Breakfast Quinoa 16
  - Jamaican Cornmeal Porridge 16
  - Breakfast Green Chile 16
  - French Toast Casserole 16
  - Instant Pot Bread Pudding 17
  - Steamed Scotch Eggs 17
  - Banana French Toast 17
  - Ham, Egg, And Cheese Casserole 18
  - Instant Pot Hard Boiled Eggs 18
  - Instant Pot Breakfast Coconut Yogurt 18
  - Crustless And Meaty Quiche 18
  - Apple Delicata Squash Porridge 18
  - Vegan Pumpkin Coffee Cake Oatmeal 19
  - Potato Egg Frittata 19
  - Extra Thick Almond Milk Yogurt 19
  - Blueberry Breakfast Oats 19
  - Instant Pot Banana Bread 20
  - Egg and Broccoli Casserole 20
  - Blueberry French Toast 20
- Delicious Egg Recipes 21
  - Instant Pot Egg Cups 21
  - Instant Pot Egg Muffins 21
  - Instant Pot Breakfast Frittatas 21
  - Basic Instant Pot Egg Salad Recipe 21
  - Instant Pot Perfectly Soft-Boiled Eggs 21
  - Sous Vide Egg Bites 21
  - Instant Pot Scrambled Eggs 22
  - Instant Pot Egg Custard 22
  - Instant Pot Eggs in Marinara Sauce 22
  - Indian Scrambled Eggs 22
  - Eggs and Chorizo 23
  - Asian Scrambled Eggs 23
  - Instant Pot Poblano Cheese Frittata 23
  - Herbed Crustless Quiche 23
  - Asparagus and Chive Frittata 24
  - Sausage, Ham, And Cheese Quiche 24
  - Bacon and Broccoli Quiche 24
  - Instant Pot Southwest Biscuit Egg Bake 25
  - Easy Instant Pot Poached Eggs 25
  - Instant Pot Hong Kong Egg Custard 25
  - Cheesy Egg Casserole 25
  - Instant Pot Deviled Eggs 25
  - Instant Pot Lemon Orzo Soup 26
  - Instant Pot Hard Boiled Egg Loaf 26
  - Instant Pot Bacon and Broccoli Frittata 26
  - Turkey Egg Breakfast Casserole 26
  - Simple Egg Casserole 27
  - Potato Bacon Egg Breakfast 27
  - Sausages and Eggs 27
  - 5-Ingredient Shakshuka 27
  - Pepperoni and Potato Frittata 28
  - Zucchini and Eggs 28
  - Silver Beet and Dukkah Baked Eggs 28
  - Chives and Eggs Casserole 28
  - Spinach Baked Eggs with Parmesan on Toast . 29
  - One-Pan Eggs and Peppers 29
  - Instant Pot Coddled Eggs 29
  - Baked Eggs with Chorizo 29
  - Romesco Eggs with Sausages 30
  - Egg Masala Curry 30
  - Eggs in Pots with Smoked Salmon Casserole .. 30
  - Toad-in-the-hole Eggs and Tomatoes 30
  - Simple Savory Tomatoes and Eggs 31
  - Chorizo, Kale and Apple Frittata 31
  - Mexican Eggs with Potato Hash 31
- Beans Recipes 32
  - Pinto Beans with Chorizo 32
  - Simple Boiled Pinto Beans 32
  - Simple Boiled Kidney Beans 32
  - Black Eyed Peas and Ham 32
  - Simple Spiced Black Beans 32
  - Instant Pot Easy Baked Beans 32
  - Greek Gigante Beans 33
  - 15-Bean Soup 33
  - Instant Pot Refried Beans 33
  - 13-Bean Soup 33
  - Lazy Man's Baked Beans 33
  - Easy Lazy Pressure Cooker Chili 34
  - Pumpkin Lentil Soup 34
  - Instant Pot Green Split Pea Soup 34
  - 15-Bean Tailgate Chili in Instant Pot 34
  - Instant Pot Hummus 35
  - Instant Pot Red Beans and Rice 35
  - Instant Pot Ham and Bean Soup 35

Instant Pot Drunken Beans 35
Tex-Mex Pinto Beans 35
Beans with Cajun Sausages Soup 36
Sweet and Savory Baked Beans 36
Instant Pot Cuban Black Beans 36
Indian Green Beans and Potatoes 36
Brothy Beans with Cream 37
Navy Bean Escarole Stew 37
Sausage Greens and Bean Pasta 37
Cannellini Beans with Shrimp and Tomatoes 37
Spice Bean and Chicken Chorizo Chili 38
Mixed Beans Salad 38
Black Bean Soup with Poblano Chilies 38
Butter Bean Ragout 38
Spicy Beans with Wilted Greens 39
Cannellini Beans Stew with Chicken and Dried Cherries 39
Cannellini and Tomato Soup 39
Spicy Bean Soup with Sausages 40
Pasta Cannellini with Escarole 40
Mexican Beans with Beef Soup 40
Gigante Beans in Tomato Sauce 40
Baked with Beans with Bacon 41
Spicy Fava Bean Soup 41
Beans and Squash Minestrone 41
White Beans and Broccoli 41
Italian Bean Stew 42
Stewed Spicy Cannellini Beans 42
Grains Recipes 43
Instant Pot Rice 43
Chicken and Rice 43
Indian Vegetable Rice 43
Cilantro Lime Rice 43
Instant Pot Spanish Rice 43
Instant Pot Rice Pilaf 44
Instant Pot Ground Beef Shawarma Rice 44
Instant Pot Cajun Chicken and Rice 44
Hibachi Fried Rice 44
Instant Pot Mexican Rice 45
Instant Pot Creamy Mushroom Wild Rice Soup 45
Rice with Chicken and Broccoli 45
Instant Pot Mushroom Risotto 45
Basic Instant Pot Risotto 46
Instant Pot Porcini Risotto 46
Risotto with Bacon and Peas 46
Instant Pot Asparagus Risotto 46
Butternut Squash Risotto 47
Spinach and Goat Cheese Risotto 47
Roasted Cauliflower Barley Risotto 47
Instant Pot Pearl Barley 47
Pearl Barley Soup 48
Chicken Barley Soup 48
Beef Barley Soup 48
Beefy Instant Pot Congee 48
Vietnamese Chicken Congee (Chao Ga) 48
Instant Pot Basic Congee (Jook) 49
Brown Rice Congee with Shiitake Mushrooms49
Festive Chicken Ginger Congee 49
Instant Pot Buckwheat Porridge 49

Basic Instant Pot Quinoa 49
One-Minute Quinoa and Veggies 50
Mexican Quinoa with Cilantro Sauce 50
Quinoa Fried Rice 50
Instant Pot Quinoa Pilaf 50
Quinoa with Mushrooms and Vegetables 51
Basic Instant Pot Millet 51
Instant Pot Millet Porridge 51
Creamy Millet Breakfast Porridge 51
Proofing Whole Wheat Bread in Instant Pot .. 51
Instant Pot Coconut Oatmeal 52
Banana Walnut Steel-Cut Oats 52
Instant Pot Apple Spice Oats 52
Pumpkin Spice Oat Meal 52
Peaches and Cream Oatmeal 52
Chicken Recipes 53
Lemon Olive Chicken 53
Italian Chicken Marsala 53
Instant Pot Chicken Cacciatore 53
Honey Bourbon Chicken 53
Butter Chicken Murgh Makhani 53
Honey Sesame Chicken 54
Instant Pot Rotisserie Chicken 54
Instant Pot Shredded Chicken 54
Instant Pot Mongolian Chicken 54
Instant Pot Chicken Adobo 55
Moringa Chicken Soup 55
Lemon Mustard Chicken with Potatoes 55
Lemongrass and Coconut Chicken 55
Instant Pot Crack Chicken 55
Instant Pot Chicken Biryani 56
Smokey Honey Cilantro Chicken 56
Thai Chicken Stew 56
Chili Lime Chicken 56
Honey Teriyaki Chicken 57
Instant Pot Cashew Chicken 57
40-Clove Chicken 57
Instant Pot BBQ Chicken with Potatoes 57
Asian Garlic and Honey Chicken 58
Mojo Chicken Tacos 58
Instant Pot Orange Chicken 58
Belizean Stewed Chicken 58
Lazy Sweet and Sour Chicken 59
Chicken with White Wine Mushroom Sauce .. 59
Instant Pot Jamaican Jerk Chicken 59
Instant Pot Chicken Creole 59
Instant Pot Chicken Piccata 60
Root Beer Chicken Wings 60
Instant Pot Alfredo Chicken Noodles 60
Chicken with Mushrooms and Mustard 60
Quick Hoisin Chicken 61
Sticky Chicken and Chilies 61
Instant Pot Herbed Chicken 61
Yakitori Chicken Wings 61
Balsamic Orange Chicken Drumsticks 61
French Style Chicken Potatoes 62
Stocks and Sauces Recipes 63
Basic Vegetable Stock 63
Turkey Giblet Stock 63
Basic Beef Stock 63

Asian Chicken Stock 63
Simple Bone Broth 63
Japanese Dashi Stock 64
Instant Pot Scotch Broth 64
Smoked Turkey Stock 64
Instant Pot White Stock 64
Hoshi Shiitake Dashi 64
Vegan and Gluten-Free Stock 64
Mushroom Gravy Sauce 65
Asian Soup Stock 65
Turkey Soup Stock 65
Thai Soup Stock 65
Chinese Pork Stock 66
Classic Pork Broth 66
Seafood Soup Stock 66
Easy Venison Broth 66
Instant Pot Herb Stock 66
Korean-Style Dashi Stock 67
Vietnamese Pho Stock 67
Roasted Chicken Stock 67
Magic Mineral Broth 67
Instant Pot Shellfish Stock 68
Instant Pot Cranberry Sauce 68
Instant Pot Strawberry Applesauce 68
Instant Pot Mushroom Broth 68
Chicken Feet Stock 68
Vegan Beef Stock 69
Instant Pot Ham Bone Broth 69
10-Minute Mushroom Broth 69
Chinese Master Stock 69
Vegan Chicken Stock 69
Browned Chicken Broth 70
Classic Chicken Bone Broth 70
Leftover Turkey Carcass Soup 70
3-Ingredient Bone Broth 70
Easy Savory Turkey Stock 71
Classic Beef Bone Broth 71

Soups, Stews, and Chilies Recipes 72
Cuban Black Bean Soup 72
Garden Harvest Soup 72
Whole Food Minestrone Soup 72
Instant Pot Football Chili 72
Beef Borscht Soup 72
Chicken and Sweet Potato Chipotle Soup 73
Swiss Chard Stem Soup 73
Instant Pot Chicken Tortilla Soup 73
Instant Pot Cheddar, Broccoli, And Potato Soup 73
Instant Pot Lasagna Soup 74
Chicken Faux Pho 74
Ethiopian Spinach and Lentil Soup 74
Mexican Meatball Soup 75
Hearty and Creamy Broccoli Soup 75
Butternut and Cauliflower Stew 75
Instant Pot Cheeseburger Soup 75
Instant Pot Zuppa Toscana 75
Creamy Thai Coconut Chicken Soup 76
Red Lentil Chili 76
Instant Pot Pork Vindaloo 76
Instant Pot Goat Stew 76

Instant Pot Kimchi Stew (Korean Kimchi Jjigae) 77
Puchero A La Valencia (Spanish Stew) 77
Instant Pot Ham and Potato Soup 77
Easy Corn Chowder 78
Beans and Tomato Stew 78
African Peanut Butter Beef Stew 78
Italian Sausage Stew 78
Enchilada Chicken Stew 79
Instant Pot Goulash 79
Instant Pot Carne Guisada 79
Instant Pot Turkey Chili 79
Classic Beef Chili 80
Instant Pot Chipotle Chili 80
Instant Pot Cowboy Chili 80
Instant Pot Green Chili Stew 80
Texas Beef Chili 81
White Chicken Chili 81
Instant Pot Turkey Chili 81
Cheesy Chili Mac 81
Salmon and Veggies 82
Salmon and Rice Pilaf 82
Instant Pot Poached Salmon 82
Spicy Lemon Halibut 82
Instant Pot Salmon Fillet 83
Simple Instant Pot Salmon 83
Salmon with Lemon Caper Chimichurri 83
Asian Fish and Vegetables 83
Instant Pot Mediterranean Fish 83
Thai Coconut Fish 84
Fish with Orange and Ginger Sauce 84
Fish Coconut Curry 84
Green Chili Mahi Mahi 84
Wild Alaskan Cod 84
Old Bay Fish Tacos 84
Instant Pot Mok Pa 85
Chinese-Style Steamed Ginger Scallion Fish 85
Sweet and Spicy Mahi Mahi 85
Lemon and Dill Fish Packets 85
Instant Pot Shrimps 86
Instant Pot Shrimp Boil 86
Instant Pot Jambalaya 86
Shrimps in Lobsters Sauce 86
Crabs in Coconut Milk 86
Steamed Shrimps and Asparagus in Instant Pot 87
Instant Pot Seafood Stew 87
Japanese Seafood Curry 87
Clams and Corn 87
Steamed Crab Legs 87
Lobster with Wine and Tomatoes 88
Instant Pot Mussels 88
Instant Pot Boiled Octopus 88
Instant Pot Lobster Roll 88
Instant Pot Easy Scallops 88
Instant Pot Tuna Casserole 89
Lemon Shrimps with Veggies and Parmesan 89
Mediterranean-Style Cod 89
Coconut Curry Sea Bass 89
Creamy Haddock with Kale 89

Steamed Fish Patra Ni Maachi 90
Asian Pot Roast 90
Italian Pot Roast 90
Simple Instant Pot Roast 90
Classic Pot Roast 91
Sunday Pot Roast 91
Balsamic Pot Roast 91
Instant Pot Beef Mechado 91
Greek Style Beef Stew 91
Mississippi Coke Beef 92
Instant Pot Cheese Steak 92
Instant Pot Sauerbraten (German-Style Beef) 92
Chunky and Beanless Beef Chili 92
BBQ Beef Ribs 93
Mocha-Rubbed Roast 93
Poor Man's Pot Roast 93
Italian Short Ribs 93
Korean Short Ribs 93
Basic Braised Beef Short Ribs 94
Asian Short Ribs 94
Simple Bone-In Ribs 94
Irish Beef Stew 94
Instant Pot Beef Burgundy 94
Sweet and Smoky Short Ribs 95
Mexican Short Ribs 95
Korean Style Galbijjm 95
Vietnamese Beef Bo Kho 95
Vegetable Beef Stew 95
Five Spice Beef Stew 96
Mole Beef Stew 96
Instant Pot Carne Guisada 96
Instant Pot Nikujaga 96
Brazilian Beef Stew (Feijoada) 97
Beef Barley Stew with Sour Cream 97
Instant Pot Mongolian Beef 97
Easy Beef and Broccoli Stir Fry 97
Instant Pot Beef Ragu 98
Italian Tomato Meatballs 98
Instant Pot Sloppy Joes 98
Korean Basil Beef Bowls 98
Corned Beef Brisket 99
Pork Recipes 100
Instant Pot Ribs 100
Smoky BBQ Instant Pot Ribs 100
Sticky Glazed Spare Ribs 100
Coffee Pork Ribs 100
Instant Pot Korean Glazed Ribs 100
Maple Spice Rubbed Ribs 100
Sweet and Sour Riblets 101
Fall-Of-The-Bones Ribs 101
Greek Pork Ribs 101
Instant Pot Barbecue Ribs 101
Instant Pot Kalua Pig 101
Western Shoulder Ribs 101
Pork Ribs with Memphis Rub 102
Instant Pot Paleo Carnitas 102
Smoked Pull Pork 102
BBQ Pulled Pork 102
Orange-Glazed Pork Chops 102
Buffalo Pork Chops 103
Honey Lime Ginger Pork Chops 103
Instant Pot Pork Adobo 103
Instant Pot Curried Pork Chops 103
Pork Chops with Honey Mustard 103
Smothered Pork Chops 104
Chili Verde Recipe 104
Instant Pot Pineapple Ham 104
Beer-Braised Pulled Ham 104
Cranberry Maple Orange Pork Chops 104
3-Ingredient Pork Chops 105
Shortcut Pork Posole 105
Moo Shu Pork 105
Instant Pot Asian Pork Belly 105
Instant Pot Pork Stroganoff 105
Hungarian Pork Paprikash 106
Simple General Tso's Pork 106
Peppercorn Pork Brisket 106
Ginger Pork Shogayaki 106
Chile Pork Stew 106
Chinese BBQ Pork (Char Siu) 107
Balsamic Spiced Apple Pork 107
Sweet Chili Sauce Braised Pork 107
Vegetables and Sides Recipes 108
Instant Pot Cauliflower Soup 108
Instant Pot Cauliflower Curry 108
Curried Squash Stew 108
Vegan Pumpkin Stew 108
Instant Pot Vegan Stroganoff 108
Tomato and Basil Soup 108
Instant Pot Easy Mushroom Chili 109
Crockpot Pumpkin Chili 109
Vegan Pulled "Pork" 109
Instant Pot Cajun Peanuts 109
Indian Coconut Kale Curry 109
Veggie Cheese Soup 109
Instant Pot Zucchini Casserole 110
Creamy Artichoke, Garlic, And Zucchini 110
Crockpot Summer Veggies Side Dish 110
Instant Pot Basic Steamed Vegetables 110
Instant Pot French Onion Soup 110
Steamed Vegetables Side Dish 111
Vegan Miso Risotto 111
Farro And Cherry Salad 111
Savory Mashed Sweet Potatoes 111
Sun-Dried Tomato Polenta 112
Spicy Thai Quinoa Salad 112
Rice Pilaf with Vegetables 112
Grains and Kale Salad 112
Pressure Cooker Mashed Potatoes 113
Aromatic Rosemary Garlic Potatoes 113
Simple Green Beans Salad 113
Creamy Cheese Au Gratin 113
Sweet Sticky Carrots 113
Brussels Sprouts With Pine Nuts and
Pomegranate Seeds 114
Smoking Hot Pickled Green Chilies 114
Simple Pressure Cooker Chickpea Hummus 114
Simple Eggplant Spread 114
Steamed Savory Artichokes 115
Creamy Bean and Artichoke Dip 115

Recipe	Page
Instant Pot Steamed Artichoke	115
Asian Sesame Noodles	115
Simple Rice Salad	115
Spicy Brown Rice Salad with Black Beans	116
Sweet Apple Pudding	116
Instant Pot "Baked" Apples	116
Instant Pot Oreo Cheesecake	116
Asian Coconut Rice Pudding	117
Instant Pot Crème Brule	117
Pumpkin and Rice Pudding	117
Steamed Cranberry Pudding	117
Sweet Coconut Tapioca	118
Steamed Key Lime Pie	118
Dulce De Leche	118
Fast Pressure Cooker Hazelnut Flan	118
Steamed Carrot Pudding Cake	119
Coconut Pina Colada Pudding	119
Pumpkin and Chocolate Bundt Cake	119
Instant Pot Cherry Compote	120
Steamed Keto Chocolate Cake	120
Instant Pot Raspberry Curd	120
Steamed Lemon Cake	120
Instant Pot Chocolate Lava Cake	120
Mocha Pudding Cake	121
Instant Pot Basic Steamed Vanilla Cake	121
Steamed Dark Chocolate Cake	121
Cinnamon Blondie Pecan Bars	121
Pumpkin Pie Pudding	122
Easy Instant Pot Cheesecake	122
Apple Streusel Dessert	122
Hot Fudge Sundae Cake	122
Cranberry Stuffed Apples	123
Gingerbread Pudding Cake	123
Slow Cooker Berry Cobbler	123
Pink Grapefruit Cheesecake	124
Maple Crème Brulee	124
Sweet Rice Pudding	124
Coconut, Cranberry, And Quinoa Crockpot Breakfast	124
Caramel and Pear Pudding	124
Double Dark Chocolate Cake	125
Apple Cinnamon Cake	125
Fruit Salad Jam	125
Pumpkin Spice Chocolate Chip Cookies	125
Instant Pot Sweetened Rhubarb	126
Appendix : Recipes Index	127

Introduction
The Benefits of The Instant Pot

The Instant Pot is one of the niftiest kitchen gadgets that you will ever need. There are so many benefits that you can get from using this device. Let's explore the wonderful benefits of the Instant Pot to convince you to get one today–that is, if you are still contemplating on buying one.

- Saves time and energy: Since Instant Pot is a digital pressure cooker, you can cook food faster than on the stove top. In fact, you can cook food 70% faster using the Instant Pot. This is also equated to savings in your electrical bills because you use less energy to cook your food.
- Convenient cooking: You can dump ingredients in the Instant Pot, turn it on, and wait for it to cook. The thing is that you can reduce the preparation time significantly so that you can spend more time doing more important things instead of slaving in the kitchen.
- Preserves nutrients: Cooking with a pressure cooker involves the use of heat evenly distributed inside the pressure cooker. You also do not need to use a lot of water as it generates steam to cook food. Because you are cooking food in a sealed environment, the vitamins and minerals are not lost by water or steam. Moreover, the absence of air lessens the oxidation rates of the ingredients, so the vegetables are cooked yet still retain their vibrant color compared to cooking on stove top.
- Mess-free cooking: Instant Pots come with sealed cooking mechanisms thus no steam and smell can spread out in your entire home during the cooking time. Thus, you can enjoy a mess-free cooking experience with this kitchen device.
- Cooks while sterilizing food: Many types of food contain natural toxins. For instance, rice and peanuts carry aflatoxins from molds that can cause liver cancer but can be destroyed by high heat. Because food is cooked at temperatures that are higher than the boiling point, you can also sterilize your food while cooking at the same time.
- More functional settings: Unlike other kitchen gadgets, the Instant Pot provides many functional settings, so you don't need to buy different kitchen devices to cook different types of food. The thing is that you can cook rice, ferment yogurt, and cook tough pieces of meats in one pot.

How to Use the Instant Pot?

Using the Instant Pot is not rocket science. Although it comes with a lot of buttons, you can easily use it because of its intuitive control panel and buttons. Thus, this chapter is dedicated to teaching you how to use the Instant Pot from start to finish.

Unboxing Your Instant Pot

Unboxing your Instant Pot can be an exciting thing. To make sure that your Instant Pot will work efficiently, it is crucial that you unbox it carefully and run some tests before you start cooking with it. Below are the steps on how to unbox your Instant Pot so that you can start making your favorite comfort foods with it.

- Remove all plastic film coverings: When unboxing the Instant Pot, make sure that you remove the plastic film that covers the entire Instant Pot.
- Remove the lid: Turn the lid counter-clockwise to remove it. The Instant Pot also comes with arrow indicators on the lid so that you know where to turn to close or open it. Once you open the lid remove the tools that are included in the Instant Pot such as the electric plug, cups, and other accessories.
- Attach the condensation cup: The condensation cup is a rectangular plastic cup that collects any liquid or steam that formed on the vents. This will keep the exterior of your pot as well as your kitchen mess-free.
- Check the weight knob on the lid: The weighted knob is located on top of the lid and it allows you to seal or open the vents. If you are cooking under high pressure, make sure that the knob is set to the "sealing" mode.
- Check the pressure pin: To be able to achieve high pressure, the pressure cooker needs to have a pressure pin. This tiny metal allows the pressure cooker to release pressure if there is too much inside the pot. The pressure pin should be free from any dirt so that it does not release too much heat and pressure from inside the pot.
- Check the sealing ring: The sealing ring is made from heat-tolerant rubber and, as the name implies, it seals off the lid and prevents pressure from escaping. The presence of damages and nicks on the sealing ring makes the lid less efficient in building a highly pressurized environment in the pot so you end up cooking your food longer as you would on ordinary stovetop methods.
- Insert the power cord: The power cord can be inserted on the back. Make sure that it is secured to prevent any problems in the future. Once you have inserted the cord, plug the Instant Pot into a powder source.
- Run a steam test: Running a steam test is crucial so that you can be assured that your Instant Pot is working properly. To do a steam test, fill the inner pot with water. Close the lid and seal the vent. Press the Steam button and adjust the time to 2 minutes. The Instant Pot should not release any steam during the entire steam test.

How to Cook with Your Instant Pot

Cooking food in your Instant Pot is very easy. Once you are done testing your Instant Pot, you can start cooking your favorite recipes. While there are many cooking methods that you can do with the Instant Pot, below are great cooking tips to optimize the use of this nifty kitchen device.

- Always open the lid when you opt for the Sauté option: When choosing the Sauté button, make sure that the lid is off from the Instant Pot so that you can stir your ingredients well.
- Use at the minimum ½ cup water: You don't need a lot of water to cook your food as the Instant Pot generates steam from whatever amount of water included in the recipe. In fact, you only need at least ½ cup of water to generate enough steam to cook your food.
- Reduce cooking time of recipes cooked using traditional cooking methods: If you want to cook your favorite food in the Instant Pot but you are following conventional cooking methods, reduce the cooking time of your recipes when using the Instant Pot instead
- Never use the delay timer when cooking meats: Do not use the delay timer when cooking meats because the meat may go rancid if not cooked immediately. You can only use this method if you are cooking grains or beans as they take a longer time to go rancid.
- Release the pressure carefully: Once the food is cooked, the pressure cooker needs to release the pressure inside so that the pot can be opened. There are two ways to release pressure carefully and these include the natural and quick pressure release. Natural pressure release allows the pressure cooker to release the pressure on its own accord while quick pressure release allows you to release the pressure by setting the valve from "sealing" to "venting". When doing quick pressure release, make sure that the steam vent is away from you so that you don't get burned from the escaping steam.

Instant Pot FAQs

Q1: Is it easy to cook using the Instant Pot?
Answer: There is always a learning curve when it comes to cooking with pressure cookers specifically the Instant Pot. But do not worry as once you are familiar with it, cooking with the Instant Pot becomes really easy

Q2: Is it safe to use?
Answer: The Instant Pot is quiet and very safe to use. It has a 10 UL Certified safety mechanism to prevent any potential issues.

Q3: What is the Instant Pot's working pressure?
Answer: The Instant Pot has a working pressure of 10.15 to 11.6 PSI.

Q4: Can it be used for pressure canning?
Answer: While theoretically, pressure cookers can be used for canning, the official website of Instant Pot noted that the "Instant Pot has not been tested for food safety in pressure canning by USDA. The programs in Instant Pot are regulated by a pressure sensor instead of a thermometer, the elevation of where you live can also affect the cooking temperature. For now, we wouldn't recommend using Instant Pot for pressure canning purpose."

Q5: Can I use it for pressure frying?
Answer: Never attempt to do pressure frying with electrical pressure cookers including Instant Pot. The splattering oil can melt the gasket and can damage the entire device.

Q6: How to do quick pressure release?
Answer: After the cooking cycle ends to move the venting knob from the sealing to the venting position. This will rapidly release the pressure from inside the inner pot. Wait until the floating valve drops before you open the lid.

Q7: I live in a high-altitude place. Do I need to adjust the cooking time?
Answer: The altitude can affect the cooking settings and time of the pressure cooker. Most of the recipes developed for Instant Pot are tested at close to the sea level. So, if you live over 3000 feet above sea level, adjust the cooking time to longer.

Mouthwatering Breakfast Recipes

Sweet Potato Hash

Serves: 6
Preparation Time: 5 minutes
Cooking Time: 15 minutes

Ingredients
- 1 large sweet potatoes, scrubbed and sliced
- 3 cups butternut squash, cubed
- 1 cup water
- 2 tablespoons butter
- 4 cloves of garlic, minced
- ½ onion, sliced
- 1 teaspoon salt
- 1 teaspoon thyme
- 1 teaspoon parsley

Instructions
1. Place the sweet potatoes and butternut squash slices into the Instant Pot.
2. Pour in the water and close the lid. Press the Manual button and cook for 10 minutes.
3. Do quick pressure release and drain the water.
4. Transfer the sweet potatoes and butternut squash into a bowl.
5. Without the lid on press the Sauté button and add the butter. Sauté the garlic and onion.
6. Add the sweet potatoes and butternut squash. Season with salt, thyme, and parsley.
7. Continue sautéing for 5 minutes

Nutrition information:
Calories per serving: 96; Carbohydrates: 15.8g; Protein: 1.5g; Fat: 3.9g; Fiber: 3.5g

Saucy Spanish Chorizo and Potato Hash

Serves: 7
Preparation Time: 5 minutes
Cooking Time: 15 minutes

Ingredients
- 1 tablespoon olive oil
- 1 tablespoon minced garlic
- 1 onion, diced
- 6 large potatoes, peeled and wedges
- 1 chorizo sausage, sliced
- 4 slices of bacon, chopped
- 1 cup cream cheese
- ½ cup Greek yogurt
- ½ cup vegetable stock
- 3 tablespoons rosemary
- Salt and pepper to taste

Instructions
1. Without the lid on, press the Sauté button on the Instant Pot.
2. Add the oil and sauté the garlic and onion for a few minutes.
3. Stir in the potatoes, bacon, and sausages. Continue cooking for three more minutes.
4. Add the rest of the ingredients. Give a stir.
5. Close the lid and select the Manual button.
6. Adjust the cooking time to 10 minutes.
7. Do natural pressure release.

Nutrition information:
Calories per serving: 578; Carbohydrates: 59.6g; Protein: 11.83g; Fat: 34.2g; Fiber: 7.6g

Bacon Ranch Potatoes

Serves: 6
Preparation Time: 3 minutes
Cooking Time: 7 minutes

Ingredients
- 2 pounds red potatoes, scrubbed clean and cut into wedges
- 3 bacon strips, chopped
- 2 teaspoons dried parsley
- 1 teaspoon salt
- 1 teaspoon garlic powder
- 1 cup cheddar cheese, grated
- 1/3 cup Ranch dressing

Instructions
1. Add all ingredients except for the cheddar cheese and Ranch dressing into the Instant Pot.
2. Stir to combine all ingredients
3. Close the lid and seal off the vent.
4. Press the Manual button and adjust the cooking time to 7 minutes.
5. Cook under high pressure and allow to naturally release the pressure.
6. Open the lid and stir in the cheese and Ranch dressing.

Nutrition information:
Calories per serving: 337; Carbohydrates: 35.5g; Protein: 16.1g; Fat: 15.2g; Fiber: 2.7g

Loaded Breakfast Potatoes

Serves: 4
Preparation Time: 10 minutes
Cooking Time: 20 minutes

Ingredients
- 4 russet potatoes, scrubbed
- 1-pound pork sausage, chopped
- ¼ cup onion, diced
- 1 red bell pepper, diced
- 1 orange bell pepper, diced
- ½ teaspoon garlic powder
- Salt and pepper to taste

Instructions
1. Place the steamer rack in the Instant Pot and pour a cup of water.
2. Place the potatoes on the rack.
3. Close the lid and seal off the valve.
4. Press the Manual button and adjust the cooking time to 20 minutes.
5. Meanwhile, heat a skillet and place the pork sausage slices until the fat has slightly rendered.
6. Add the rest of the vegetables and season with garlic powder, salt, and pepper to taste.
7. Once the Instant Pot is done cooking the potatoes, take the potatoes out and place on a plate.
8. Pour over the sausage and vegetable mixture.

Nutrition information:

Calories per serving: 570; Carbohydrates: 73.8g; Protein: 20.6g; Fat: 22.4g; Fiber: 5.5g

Cheesy Egg Bake

Serves: 6
Preparation Time: 5 minutes
Cooking Time: 8 minutes
Ingredients
- 6 eggs, beaten
- ¼ cup milk
- 1 teaspoon salt
- ½ teaspoon pepper
- 6 slices of bacon, chopped
- 2 cups hash browns
- 1 cup spinach
- ½ cup button mushrooms, sliced
- ½ cup cheddar cheese, grated

Instructions
1. In a mixing bowl, combine the eggs and milk. Season with salt and pepper to taste. Beat until well combined then set aside.
2. Press the Sauté button on the Instant Pot and add the bacon. Cook the bacon until some of the fat has rendered. Set aside.
3. Arrange the hash browns at the bottom of the Instant Pot and add the bacon, spinach, and mushrooms.
4. Pour over the egg mixture.
5. Top with grated cheese.
6. Close the lid and press the Manual button. Cook on high for 8 minutes or until the eggs are cooked through.
7. Do natural pressure release.

Nutrition information:
Calories per serving:354; Carbohydrates: 16.5g; Protein: 14.1g; Fat: 26.9g; Fiber: 1.8g

Lemon Blueberry Breakfast Cake

Serves: 6
Preparation Time: 15 minutes
Cooking Time: 30 minutes
Ingredients
- 2 cups all-purpose flour
- 2 teaspoon baking powder
- ½ teaspoon salt
- 1 lemon, zested
- ¾ cup sugar
- ½ cup unsalted butter, at room temperature
- 1 egg, at room temperature
- 1 teaspoon vanilla extract
- ½ cup buttermilk
- 2 cups frozen blueberries
- ½ lemon, juiced freshly squeezed
- ½ cup powdered sugar for dusting

Instructions
1. Get a heat-proof baking dish that will fit in the Instant Pot. Grease and flour, it and set aside.
2. Pour a cup of water into the Instant Pot. Set aside and prepare the cake.
3. In a mixing bowl, combine the flour, baking soda, and salt until well-combined.
4. Add the zest, sugar, and butter.
5. Use a mixer and beat until the entire ingredients are combined.
6. Add the egg and vanilla extract. Gradually add the buttermilk and continue mixing until combined.
7. Toss the blueberries into the batter.
8. Pour the batter into the greased pans until it is ¾ full. Place aluminum foil on top.
9. Place inside the Instant Pot and close the lid.
10. Press the Manual button and cook for 30 minutes.
11. Do natural pressure release.
12. Dust with powdered sugar before serving.

Nutrition information:
Calories per serving:388; Carbohydrates: 61.7g; Protein: 7.4g; Fat:12.9 g; Fiber: 2.6g

Bacon and Cheese Crustless Quiche

Serves: 6
Preparation Time: 5 minutes
Cooking Time: 10 minutes
Ingredients
- 6 eggs, lightly beaten
- 1 cup milk
- Salt and pepper to taste
- 2 cups Monterey Jack cheese, grated
- 1 cup bacon, cooked and crumbled

Instructions
1. Spray the inner pot of the Instant Pot with cooking spray.
2. In a mixing bowl, mix together the eggs, milk, salt, and pepper until well-combined.
3. Place the bacon and cheese in the Instant Pot and pour over the egg mixture.
4. Close the lid and press the Manual button. Adjust the cooking time to 10 minutes.
5. Do natural pressure release.

Nutrition information:
Calories per serving: 396; Carbohydrates: 5.5g; Protein: 23.7g; Fat: 31.3g; Fiber: 0.7g

Eggs Benedict Casserole

Serves: 6
Preparation Time: 10 minutes
Cooking Time: 10 minutes
Ingredients
- 1 tablespoon olive oil
- 6 large eggs, beaten
- 2 ½ cups milk
- 1 ½ teaspoon dried mustard
- 1 ½ cup heavy cream
- 6 English muffins, cubed
- 1 leek, chopped
- 1 cup bacon, cooked and crumbled
- 2 tablespoons chives
- ½ teaspoon cayenne pepper
- 1 stick butter
- 8 egg yolks, at room temperature
- 1 tablespoon lemon juice
- 1 teaspoon Dijon mustard
- ½ cup heavy cream
- ½ teaspoon salt
- ¼ teaspoon black pepper

Instructions
1. Grease the Instant Pot with olive oil.

2. In a mixing bowl, mix together the eggs, milk, dried mustard, and heavy cream until well-combined. Set aside.
3. Place the English muffins in the Instant Pot. Add the leeks, bacon, chives, and cayenne pepper.
4. Pour over the egg mixture.
5. Close the lid and seal off the vent. Press the Manual button and adjust the cooking time to 10 minutes.
6. Meanwhile, prepare the hollandaise sauce by combining all ingredients in a bowl. Place the bowl over a double boiler and continue whisking until the mixture is thick enough to coat the back of the spoon.
7. Once the Instant Pot is done cooking the casserole, do natural pressure release.
8. Drizzle with the hollandaise sauce before serving.
Nutrition information:
Calories per serving: 314; Carbohydrates: 15g; Protein: 21g; Fat: 20g; Fiber: 6.3g

Instant Pot Huevos Rancheros

Serves: 8
Preparation Time: 5 minutes
Cooking Time: 15 minutes
Ingredients
- 1 tablespoon butter
- 10 eggs, beaten
- 1 cup light cream
- 8 ounces Mexican blend cheese, grated
- ½ teaspoon pepper
- ¼ teaspoon chili powder
- 1 clove of garlic, crushed
- 1 can green chilies, drained
- 8 tortillas
- 1 can red enchilada sauce

Instructions
1. Grease the inside of the Instant Pot with butter.
2. In a large bowl, mix together the eggs, cream, Mexican cheese, pepper, and chili powder. Stir in the garlic and chilies.
3. Pour into the Instant Pot and close the lid. Press the Manual button and adjusts the cooking time to 15 minutes.
4. Do natural pressure release.
5. Assemble the dish by spooning the egg casserole to tortillas and serving with enchilada sauce.
Nutrition information:
Calories per serving:182; Carbohydrates: 4g; Protein: 9g; Fat: 14g; Fiber: 2.6g

Mexican-Style Quiche

Serves: 8
Preparation Time: 5 minutes
Cooking Time: 25 minutes
Ingredients
- Prepared pie crust
- 6 eggs, beaten
- ¼ teaspoon chili powder
- Salt and pepper to taste
- 4 green onions, chopped
- 1 can cannelloni beans, drained and rinsed
- 2 cups cheddar cheese, grated
- 1 cup salsa

Instructions
1. Make sure that the pie crust fits the Instant Pot.
2. Place a steamer rack in the Instant Pot and pour a cup of water.
3. In a mixing bowl, combine the eggs, chili powder, salt, and pepper.
4. Place the onion and beans in the pie crust.
5. Pour over the egg mixture and pour cheddar cheese on top. Place a foil on top.
6. Place the quiche on the steamer rack.
7. Close the lid and seal the vent.
8. Press the Steam button and adjust the cooking time to 25 minutes.
9. Do natural pressure release.
10. Serve with salsa.
Nutrition information:
Calories per serving: 318; Carbohydrates: 26.5g; Protein: 15.6g; Fat: 17.1g; Fiber: 3.7g

Easy Irish Oatmeal

Serves: 3
Preparation Time: 3 minutes
Cooking Time: 6 minutes
Ingredients
- 4 cups milk
- 1 ¾ cup steel-cut oats
- ½ cup dried cherries
- ½ cup maple syrup
- ½ teaspoon salt
- ¼ teaspoon ground allspice
- 4 cups water
- ½ cup blueberries
- 1/3 cup pecans, chopped

Instructions
1. Place all ingredients except for the pecans in the Instant Pot.
2. Give a good stir.
3. Close the lid and seal off the vents.
4. Press the Manual button and adjust the cooking time to 6 minutes.
5. Do natural pressure release.
6. Prior to serving, give the oatmeal and good stir.
7. Garnish with pecans on top.
Nutrition information:
Calories per serving: 597; Carbohydrates: 101.6g; Protein: 21.4g; Fat: 22.5g; Fiber: 10.6g

Spinach and Ham Frittata

Serves: 8
Preparation Time: 3 minutes
Cooking Time: 10 minutes
Ingredients
- 8 eggs, beaten
- 2 cloves of garlic, minced
- 2 cups spinach, chopped
- 1 cup ham, diced
- 1 onion, chopped
- ½ cup coconut milk
- 1 teaspoon salt

Instructions
1. Place all ingredients in the Instant Pot.
2. Give a good stir.
3. Close the lid and seal off the vents.

4. Press the Manual button and adjust the cooking time to 10 minutes.
5. Do natural pressure release.
Nutrition information:
Calories per serving: 63; Carbohydrates: 5g; Protein: 8g; Fat: 3g; Fiber: 2.9g

Eggs En Cocotte

Serves: 3
Preparation Time: 10 minutes
Cooking Time: 20 minutes
Ingredients
- Butter or cooking spray
- 3 tablespoons cream
- 3 eggs
- 1 tablespoon chives
- Salt and pepper to taste

Instructions
1. Place a steamer rack in the Instant Pot and pour a cup of water.
2. Grease three ramekins with butter or cooking spray.
3. Place 1 tablespoon of cream in each ramekin.
4. Carefully crack an egg into each ramekin.
5. Sprinkle with chives and season with salt and pepper on top.
6. Place on the steamer rack.
7. Close the lid and press the Manual button. Adjust the cooking time to 20 minutes.
8. Do natural pressure release.

Nutrition information:
Calories per serving: 166; Carbohydrates: 3.1g; Protein: 9.7 g; Fat: 12.7g; Fiber: 0.3g

5-Ingredient Cheesy Egg Bake

Serves: 4
Preparation Time: 5 minutes
Cooking Time: 20 minutes
Ingredients
- 6 eggs, beaten
- ¼ cup milk
- 2 cups hash browns
- 6 slices of bacon, rendered and chopped
- ½ cup cheddar cheese, grated

Instructions
1. In a mixing bowl, combine the eggs and milk until well-combined.
2. Place the hash browns in the bottom of the Instant Pot.
3. Add the bacon slices and cheddar cheese.
4. Pour over the egg mixture.
5. Close the lid and press the Manual button.
6. Adjust the cooking time to 20 minutes.
7. Do quick pressure release.

Nutrition information:
Calories per serving: 637; Carbohydrates: 30.6g; Protein: 29.2g; Fat: 44.6g; Fiber: 2.4g

Instant Pot Slow Cooker Chocolate Oatmeal

Serves: 4
Preparation Time: 5 minutes
Cooking Time: 6 hours and 30 minutes
Ingredients
- 2 cups oatmeal
- 6 cups water
- 1 cup milk
- 2 ½ tablespoons cocoa powder
- 1 teaspoon cinnamon
- 1 teaspoon vanilla
- 10 ounces cherries, frozen
- ½ cup chocolate chips, for garnish

Instructions
1. Place all ingredients except for the chocolate chips in the Instant Pot and stir.
2. Close the lid and set it on the Vent setting to use the slow cooker function.
3. Press the Slow Cooker button and cook on low for 6 ½ hours.
4. Once cooked, stir in the chocolate chips.

Nutrition information:
Calories per serving: 209; Carbohydrates: 38.8g; Protein: 6.13g; Fat: 4.7g; Fiber: 5g

Breakfast Espresso Oatmeal

Serves: 4
Preparation Time: 5 minutes
Cooking Time: 10 minutes
Ingredients
- 2 ½ cups water
- 1 cup milk
- 1 cup oats
- 2 tablespoons sugar
- 1 teaspoon espresso powder
- ¼ teaspoon salt
- 2 teaspoons vanilla extract
- A dollop of whipped cream
- 2 tablespoons grated chocolate

Instructions
1. Place all ingredients except for the whipped cream and chocolate shavings in the Instant Pot.
2. Stir to combine everything.
3. Lock the lid and close the vent.
4. Press High Pressure and set the cooking time to 10 minutes.
5. Once done, do quick pressure release
6. Serve with whip cream and sprinkle with chocolate shavings on top.

Nutrition information:
Calories per serving: 173; Carbohydrates: 35.5g; Protein: 6.4g; Fat: 5.1g; Fiber: 4g

Fruited Steel-Cut Breakfast Oats

Serves: 2
Preparation Time: 3 minutes
Cooking Time: 4 minutes
Ingredients
- 1 cup steel cut oats
- ½ cup plain Greek yogurt
- 1 ½ cup water
- 2 apples, cored and chopped
- ¼ cup maple syrup
- ½ teaspoon cloves
- ½ teaspoon cinnamon powder
- 2 tablespoons slivered almonds

Instructions

1. Place the oats in the Instant Pot.
2. Stir in the water, yogurt, apples, maple syrup, cloves, and cinnamon.
3. Close the lid and seal the valve.
4. Press the Manual button and cook for 4 minutes.
5. Do quick pressure release.
6. Stir again and garnish with slivered almonds and more maple syrup or cinnamon.
Nutrition information:
Calories per serving:330; Carbohydrates: 83.9g; Protein: 10.4g; Fat: 4.3g; Fiber: 12.1g

Trail Mix Breakfast Oatmeal

Serves: 2
Preparation Time: 5 minutes
Cooking Time: 10 minutes
Ingredients
- 1 cup steel cut oats
- 1 ½ cups water
- 2 tablespoons butter
- 1 cup orange juice, freshly squeezed
- 1 tablespoon raisins
- 1 tablespoon dried cranberries
- 1 tablespoon dried apricots, chopped
- 2 tablespoons maple syrup
- ¼ tablespoon cinnamon powder
- 2 tablespoons pecans, chopped
- A dash of salt
- ½ cup strawberries, chopped
- 1 cup granola

Instructions
1. Place in the Instant Pot all ingredients except for the strawberries and granola.
2. Close the lid and seal the vale.
3. Press the Manual button and adjust the cooking time to 10 minutes.
4. Do quick pressure release and stir the oatmeal mixture.
5. Top with strawberries and granola.
Nutrition information:
Calories per serving: 491; Carbohydrates: 76.7g; Protein: 11.5g; Fat: 24.7g; Fiber: 10.4g

Simple Breakfast Oatmeal with Brown Sugar

Serves: 2
Preparation Time: 1 minute
Cooking Time: 3 minutes
Ingredients
- 1 cup steel cut oats
- 3 cups water
- ¼ cup brown sugar, packed
- 1 tablespoon cinnamon powder

Instructions
1. Place all ingredients in the Instant Pot.
2. Give a good stir.
3. Close the lid and seal the vent.
4. Press the Manual button and adjust the cooking time to 3 minutes.
5. Do quick pressure release.
6. Stir the oatmeal and top with more brown sugar or any fruits that you desire.
Nutrition information:
Calories per serving: 230; Carbohydrates: 61.2g; Protein: 8.3g; Fat: 3.4g; Fiber:9.3g

Ham and Cheese Casserole

Serves: 8
Preparation Time: 5 minutes
Cooking Time: 10 minutes
Ingredients
- 4 medium red potatoes, sliced thinly
- ½ onion, diced
- 1 cup ham, chopped
- 10 large eggs, beaten
- 1 cup milk
- 1 teaspoon salt
- ½ teaspoon pepper
- 2 cups cheddar cheese, grated

Instructions
1. Arrange the potato slices in the Instant Pot.
2. Add the onions and chopped ham.
3. In a mixing bowl, combine the eggs and milk. Mix well and season with salt and pepper to taste.
4. Pour into the Instant Pot.
5. Top with cheddar cheese.
6. Close the lid and seal the vent.
7. Press the lid and Push the Manual button.
8. Adjust the cooking time to 10 minutes.
9. Do natural pressure release and check if the eggs are cooked through.
Nutrition information:
Calories per serving: 373; Carbohydrates: 40.3g; Protein: 22.2g; Fat: 14.2g; Fiber: 3.3g

Western Omelet Quiche

Serves: 6
Preparation Time: 5 minutes
Cooking Time: 10 minutes
Ingredients
- 6 large eggs, beaten
- ½ cup milk
- 1/8 teaspoon Himalayan salt
- 1/8 teaspoon ground black pepper
- 8 ounces bacon, chopped
- ¾ cups red and green peppers, diced
- 3 spring onions, chopped
- ¾ cup cheddar cheese, grated and divided

Instructions
1. Place all ingredients in the Instant Pot except for the half of the cheddar cheese.
2. Stir to combine everything.
3. Sprinkle with the remaining cheese on top.
4. Close the lid and seal the vent.
5. Press the Manual button and cook on high for 10 minutes or until the eggs are cooked through.
6. Do quick pressure release.
Nutrition information:
Calories per serving: 333; Carbohydrates: 17.4g; Protein: 17.6g; Fat: 22.8g; Fiber: 2.2g

French Baked Eggs

Serves: 4
Preparation Time: 10 minutes
Cooking Time: 25 minutes
Ingredients

- Olive oil for brushing
- 4 whole eggs
- 4 slices of ham
- 8 tablespoons of cream cheese
- A dash of French herb mix or any herbs of your choice
- Salt and pepper to taste

Instructions
1. Place a steam rack in the Instant Pot and pour a cup of water.
2. Brush 4 ramekins with olive oil and set aside.
3. Into each ramekin, place a slice of ham, two tablespoons of cream cheese, and a dash of mixed herbs. Crack open the eggs on each of the ramekins and season with salt and pepper to taste.
4. Place on the steam rack.
5. Close the lid and seal the vent.
6. Choose the Low pressure and adjust the cooking time to 25 minutes.
7. Do natural pressure release.

Nutrition information:
Calories per serving: 246; Carbohydrates: 3.4g; Protein: 15.2g; Fat: 19.2g; Fiber: 0.2g

Poached Eggs in Bell Pepper Cups

Serves: 2
Preparation Time: 5 minutes
Cooking Time: 10 minutes

Ingredients
- 2 fresh eggs, refrigerated
- 2 bell peppers, ends cut off and seeds removed
- 2/3 cup mayonnaise
- 1 ½ teaspoons Dijon mustard
- 3 tablespoons orange juice, freshly squeezed
- 1 tablespoon white wine vinegar
- ½ teaspoon salt
- 1 teaspoon turmeric powder
- 2 slices of whole wheat toasted bread
- 2 slices of mozzarella cheese

Instructions
1. Place a steamer basket inside the Instant Pot and add one cup of water.
2. Crack open each egg into each prepared bell pepper.
3. Wrap foil around the bell pepper and place on the steam rack.
4. Close the lid and seal the vent. Press the Manual button and select High Pressure. Adjust the cooking time to 10 minutes.
5. Once cooked, do natural pressure release.
6. Meanwhile, prepare the sauce by combining in the bowl the mayonnaise, Dijon mustard, orange juice, white wine vinegar, salt, and turmeric powder.
7. Take the bell pepper out from the Instant Pot and place on top of whole wheat bread with mozzarella cheese.
8. Drizzle with the sauce.

Nutrition information:
Calories per serving: 744; Carbohydrates: 77.3g; Protein: 26.5g; Fat: 39.8 g; Fiber: 11.1g

Mexican Egg Casserole

Serves: 8
Preparation Time: 10 minutes
Cooking Time: 20 minutes

Ingredients
- ½ cup flour
- 8 large eggs, beaten
- 1-pound sausage
- ½ onion, chopped
- 1 red bell pepper, chopped
- 1 can black beans, drained and rinsed
- ½ cup green onions
- 1 cup mozzarella cheese
- A dollop of sour cream and cilantro for garnish

Instructions
1. In a mixing bowl, combine the flour and eggs. Mix until combined then set aside.
2. Without the lid on, turn the Instant Pot and press the Sauté button.
3. Sauté the sausage and onions for about 5 minutes.
4. Pour in the egg mixture.
5. Stir in the red bell pepper, black beans, green onions, and mozzarella cheese.
6. Close the lid and seal the vent.
7. Press the Manual button and adjust the cooking time for 20 minutes.
8. Do natural pressure release.

Nutrition information:
Calories per serving:283; Carbohydrates: 19.1g; Protein: 20.6g; Fat: 15.4g; Fiber: 4.2g

Sausage and Egg Breakfast Casserole Burritos

Serves: 6
Preparation Time: 10 minutes
Cooking Time: 20 minutes

Ingredients
- 8 eggs
- 1 cup milk
- Salt and pepper to taste
- 8 ounces ground pork
- 1 teaspoon sage
- 1 teaspoon thyme
- 1 teaspoon fennel seeds, crushed
- ½ teaspoon red pepper flakes, crushed
- 1 teaspoon light brown sugar
- 1/8 teaspoon nutmeg
- 1 tablespoon water
- 6 burrito tortilla shells
- ¾ cup cheddar cheese, grated

Instructions
1. In a mixing bowl, mix the eggs and milk until well combined. Season with salt and pepper to taste.
2. Without the lid on, press the Sauté button on the Instant Pot.
3. Sauté the ground pork, sage, thyme, fennel, seeds, and red pepper flakes for 3 minutes.
4. Add the sugar, nutmeg, and water.
5. Pour in the egg mixture.
6. Close the lid and seal off the vent.
7. Press the Manual button and cook on high for 20 minutes.
8. Once cooked, serve the egg casserole into rolled tortilla shells with cheddar cheese.

Nutrition information:

Calories per serving: 454; Carbohydrates: 28.9g; Protein: 26.9g; Fat: 24.9g; Fiber: 1.6g

Yogurt with Fruits

Serves: 10
Preparation Time: 30 minutes
Cooking Time: 8 hours
Ingredients
- 1 gallon of milk
- ½ cup Greek yogurt
- 2 tablespoons vanilla bean paste
- 2 cups fruit of your own choice
- 1 cup sugar

Instructions
1. Pour the milk into the Instant Pot.
2. Close the lid and secure the vent.
3. Press the Adjust button until the display indicates "boil". This will pasteurize the milk for 45 minutes.
4. Once done, remove the inner pot from the Instant Pot and pour the milk into a clean jar. allow the milk to cook for 115 degrees Fahrenheit.
5. Clean the inner pot back into the Instant Pot and plug it in.
6. Pour in the milk, Greek yogurt, and vanilla bean paste into the Instant Pot and press the Yogurt button. The timer with reading 0:00 and adjust it to 8 hours.
7. Close the lid and allow the yogurt to ferment for 8 hours.
8. Once done, place inside clean jars and refrigerate before serving.
9. Once ready to serve, add fruits and sugar.

Nutrition information:
Calories per serving: 172; Carbohydrates: 24.6g; Protein: 3.8g; Fat: 2.3g; Fiber: 0.5g

Vanilla Apple Cinnamon Breakfast Quinoa

Serves: 2
Preparation Time: 2 minutes
Cooking Time: 8 minutes
Ingredients
- 1 cup quinoa, rinsed
- 1 ½ cups water
- ¼ teaspoon salt
- 1 apple, seeded and chopped
- 2 tablespoons cinnamon
- ½ teaspoon vanilla

Instructions
1. Add all ingredients to the Instant Pot.
2. Close the lid and seal the vent.
3. Choose the Manual button and adjust the cooking time to 8 minutes.
4. Do natural pressure release.

Nutrition information:
Calories per serving: 382; Carbohydrates: 73.5g; Protein: 12.6g; Fat: 5.4g; Fiber: 12.3g

Jamaican Cornmeal Porridge

Serves: 4
Preparation Time: 5 minutes
Cooking Time: 20 minutes
Ingredients
- 4 cups water, divided
- 1 cup yellow cornmeal
- 1 cup milk
- 2 sticks of cinnamon
- 3 pimento berries
- 1 teaspoon vanilla extract
- ½ teaspoon nutmeg, ground
- ½ cup sweetened condensed milk

Instructions
1. In a bowl, combine half of the water and cornmeal. Set aside.
2. Press the Porridge button on the Instant Pot.
3. Add the remaining water and milk into the Instant Pot. Stir in the cinnamon, pimento berries, vanilla extract, and nutmeg.
4. Pour in the cornmeal mixture then stir.
5. Close the lid and adjust the cooking time to 6 minutes.
6. Do natural pressure release.
7. Drizzle with condensed milk on top.

Nutrition information:
Calories per serving: 241; Carbohydrates: 35.8g; Protein: 5.6g; Fat: 3.8g; Fiber: 1.6g

Breakfast Green Chile

Serves: 8
Preparation Time: 5 minutes
Cooking Time: 1 hour and 30 minutes
Ingredients
- 3 pounds pork shoulder
- 1 ½ teaspoon cumin
- Salt and pepper to taste
- 3 tablespoons bacon fat
- 1 onion, chopped
- ¾ cup chicken broth
- 1 can crushed tomatoes
- 2 milk hatch green chilies
- 2 hot hatch green chilies
- 1 avocado, sliced
- Sour cream, for garnish

Instructions
1. Season the pork with cumin, salt, and pepper. Set aside.
2. Press the Sauté button on the Instant Pot and melt the bacon fat.
3. Sauté the onions and add the seasoned pork. Stir for 3 minutes then add the chicken broth, tomatoes, and chilies.
4. Close the lid and seal off the vent.
5. Press the Manual button and adjust the cooking time to 90 minutes.
6. Do quick pressure release and shred the pork using two forks.
7. Place the shredded pork into breakfast bowls and garnish with avocado slices and sour cream on top.

Nutrition information:
Calories per serving: 586; Carbohydrates: 5.3g; Protein: 48.5g; Fat: 40.3g; Fiber: 2.5g

French Toast Casserole

Serves: 6
Preparation Time: 5 minutes
Cooking Time: 15 minutes
Ingredients

- 3 eggs, beaten
- 1 cup half and half cream
- ½ cup milk
- 1 teaspoon vanilla extract
- 1 loaf French bread, cubed
- ½ cup blueberries
- 1 tablespoon cinnamon

Instructions
1. Spray the inside of the Instant Pot with cooking spray.
2. In a mixing bowl, beat the eggs with the half and half cream, and milk. Add the vanilla extract. Set aside.
3. Place the cubed French bread inside the Instant Pot.
4. Pour over the egg mixture and stir to coat the bread pieces.
5. Stir in the blueberries and sprinkle with cinnamon on top.
6. Close the lid and seal off the vent.
7. Press the Manual button and adjust the cooking time to 15 minutes.
8. Do natural pressure release.

Nutrition information:
Calories per serving: 139; Carbohydrates: 13.7g; Protein: 6.8g; Fat: 6.3g; Fiber: 1.2g

Instant Pot Bread Pudding

Serves: 12
Preparation Time: 7 minutes
Cooking Time: 15 minutes

Ingredients
- 2 cups milk
- 4 whole eggs, beaten
- ½ cup pure maple syrup
- 2 egg yolks
- 1 tablespoon vanilla extract
- ¼ teaspoon salt
- ½ cup butter, melted
- 1 loaf of bread, cubed

Instructions
1. Use a heat-proof bowl that will fit inside the Instant Pot. Grease the bowl then set aside.
2. Place a steamer rack in the Instant Pot and pour in a cup of water inside the Instant Pot. Set aside.
3. In a blender, mix together the milk, eggs, maple syrup, vanilla, and salt. Blend for 15 seconds until smooth. Add the melted butter.
4. Pour the custard mixture into the bowl and add the bread pieces. Press on the bread until all pieces get soaked with the custard mixture.
5. Place on top of the steamer rack and place aluminum foil on top.
6. Close the lid and seal the vent. Press the Steam button and adjust the cooking time to 5 minutes.
7. Do natural pressure release.
8. Allow to cool before eating.

Nutrition information:
Calories per serving:190; Carbohydrates:12.8g; Protein: 5.1g; Fat: 13.1g; Fiber: 0.1g

Steamed Scotch Eggs

Serves: 4
Preparation Time: 15 minutes
Cooking Time: 12 minutes

Ingredients
- 4 large eggs
- 1-pound ground beef
- 1 tablespoon vegetable oil

Instructions
1. Place a steamer basket in the Instant Pot and add a cup of water.
2. Place the eggs in the steamer basket and close the lid. Press the Steam button and adjust the cooking time to 6 minutes.
3. Once the timer beeps, do natural pressure release and take the eggs out. Place the eggs in an ice bath to arrest the cooking process.
4. When the eggs are cool, remove the shells. Set aside.
5. Divide the ground beef into four and flatten using your hands. Place the boiled egg in the middle and cover the entire egg with the ground beef. Do the same thing on the rest of the eggs. Set aside.
6. Press the Sauté button on the Instant Pot and add the oil. Once the oil is hot, brown the Scotch eggs on four sides. Set aside.
7. Place a steam rack in the Instant Pot and pour in a cup of water. Place the browned scotch eggs on the steamer rack and close the lid.
8. Press the Manual button and adjust the cooking time to 6 minutes.
9. Do natural pressure release.

Nutrition information:
Calories per serving:372; Carbohydrates: 0.6g; Protein: 31.3g; Fat: 26.3g; Fiber: 0g

Banana French Toast

Serves: 8
Preparation Time: 10 minutes
Cooking Time: 25 minutes

Ingredients
- 6 slices of French bread, cubed
- 4 bananas, sliced
- 2 tablespoons brown sugar
- ¼ cup cream cheese, melted in the microwave
- 3 eggs, beaten
- ½ cup milk
- 1 tablespoon white sugar
- 1 teaspoon vanilla extract
- ½ teaspoon ground cinnamon
- 2 tablespoons butter, chilled
- ¼ cup pecans, chopped

Instructions
1. Place a steamer rack in the Instant Pot and pour a cup of water.
2. Grease a baking dish that will fit in your Instant Pot. Set aside.
3. Place slices of bread into the baking dish.
4. Add a layer of banana over the bread and sprinkle with brown sugar.
5. Drizzle over the cream cheese.
6. Repeat the same layering until all ingredients are placed in the baking dish. Set aside.
7. In a mixing bowl, combine the eggs, milk, white sugar, and vanilla.

8. Pour over the baking dish and sprinkle with ground cinnamon.
9. Place the slices of butter on top and pecans.
10. Place the baking dish on the steamer rack and close the lid.
11. Press the Steam button and adjust the cooking time to 25 minutes.
12. Do natural pressure release.
Nutrition information:
Calories per serving:223; Carbohydrates: 23.3g; Protein: 6.5g; Fat: 12.1g; Fiber: 2.2g

Ham, Egg, And Cheese Casserole

Serves: 8
Preparation Time: 15 minutes
Cooking Time: 15 minutes
Ingredients
- 1 package hash browns, cubed
- 1 large onion, diced
- 2 cups ham, chopped
- 2 cups cheddar cheese, grated
- 10 large eggs, beaten
- 1 cup whole milk
- Salt and pepper to taste

Instructions
1. Spray the inside of the Instant Pot with cooking spray.
2. Place the hash browns at the bottom.
3. Arrange half of the onion, ham, and cheese. Repeat the process until all ingredients are layered into the pot.
4. In a mixing bowl, combine the eggs and milk. Season with salt and pepper.
5. Pour over the milk mixture on top of the layered ingredients.
6. Close the lid and seal off the vent.
7. Press the Manual button and cook on high for 15 minutes.
8. Do natural pressure release.
Nutrition information:
Calories per serving: 469; Carbohydrates: 30g; Protein: 33.8g; Fat: 24.1g; Fiber: 1.2g

Instant Pot Hard Boiled Eggs

Serves: 4
Preparation Time: 1 minute
Cooking Time: 8 minutes
Ingredients
- 4 eggs
- 1 cup water

Instructions
1. Pour a cup of water in the Instant Pot.
2. Place a steamer basket inside the Instant Pot.
3. Place the eggs in the steamer basket.
4. Close the lid and press the Manual button and adjust the cooking time to 8 minutes.
5. Do natural pressure release.
Nutrition information:
Calories per serving: 130; Carbohydrates: 1.2g; Protein: 8.9g; Fat: 9.6g; Fiber: 0g

Instant Pot Breakfast Coconut Yogurt

Serves: 4
Preparation Time: 20 minutes
Cooking Time: 8 hours
Ingredients
- 2 cans coconut cream
- 1 package yogurt starter
- 1 tablespoon gelatin

Instructions
1. Put the coconut cream in the Instant Pot.
2. Close the lid and seal off the vent.
3. Press the Yogurt button then the Adjust button to bring it to a boil.
4. Once the panel reads Yogurt, remove the inner pot that contains the coconut cream and place on a counter.
5. Allow the coconut cream to cool on the counter until the temperature drops to 100 0F.
6. Stir in the live culture starter until dissolved.
7. Place the inner pot back into the Instant Pot and close the lid.
8. Adjust the cooking time to 8 hours to ferment.
9. Once done, whisk in the gelatin and stir to remove the clumps.
10. Place the yogurt into clean glass jars and refrigerate for 6 hours.
Nutrition information:
Calories per serving:352; Carbohydrates: 15.2g; Protein: 6.3g; Fat: 21.9g; Fiber: 3.7g

Crustless And Meaty Quiche

Serves: 4
Preparation Time: 5 minutes
Cooking Time: 30 minutes
Ingredients
- 6 large eggs, beaten
- ½ cup milk
- Salt and pepper to taste
- 4 slices of bacon, cooked and crumbled
- 1 cup ground sausage
- ½ cup ham, diced
- 2 sprigs of green onions, chopped
- 1 cup cheddar cheese, grated

Instructions
1. Place a steamer rack in the Instant Pot and pour in a cup of water.
2. In a mixing bowl, beat the eggs and milk. Season with salt and pepper. Set aside.
3. Place the bacon, sausage, and ham in a baking dish that will fit inside the Instant Pot.
4. Pour over the egg mixture and top with green onions and cheddar cheese. Cover with aluminum foil on top.
5. Place on top of the steamer rack and close the lid.
6. Press the Steam button and cook for 30 minutes.
Nutrition information:
Calories per serving:404; Carbohydrates: 3.6g; Protein: 20.8g; Fat: 22.7g; Fiber: 1.2g

Apple Delicata Squash Porridge

Serves: 3
Preparation Time: 3 minutes
Cooking Time: 8 minutes
Ingredients
- 4 small apples, cored and diced

- 1 delicata squash, washed and cubed
- ½ cup bone broth
- 2 tablespoons maple syrup
- ½ teaspoon cinnamon
- 1/8 teaspoon cloves and ginger
- A pinch of salt

Instructions
1. Place all ingredients in the Instant Pot.
2. Close the lid and seal off the vent.
3. Press the Manual button and adjust the cooking time to 8 minutes.
4. Do natural pressure release.
5. Remove the cinnamon and cloves.
6. Place all the ingredients in a blender or use a handheld blender and pulse until smooth.

Nutrition information:
Calories per serving: 150; Carbohydrates: 39.8g; Protein: 1.3g; Fat: 0.6g; Fiber: 5.7g

Vegan Pumpkin Coffee Cake Oatmeal

Serves: 8
Preparation Time: 2 minutes
Cooking Time: 3 minutes

Ingredients
- 4 ½ cups water
- 1 ½ cups steel cut oats
- 1 ½ cups pumpkin puree
- 2 teaspoons cinnamon
- 1 teaspoon allspice
- 1 teaspoon vanilla
- ¾ cup brown sugar

Instructions
1. Place all ingredients except the brown sugar in the Instant Pot.
2. Give a good stir.
3. Close the lid and seal off the vent.
4. Press the Manual button and cook for 3 minutes.
5. Do natural pressure release.
6. Once cooked, do natural pressure release.
7. Top with brown sugar.

Nutrition information:
Calories per serving: 253; Carbohydrates: 35.9g; Protein: 9.7g; Fat: 12.3g; Fiber: 4.5g

Potato Egg Frittata

Serves: 4
Preparation Time: 5 minutes
Cooking Time: 10 minutes

Ingredients
- ¼ cup milk
- 6 large eggs, beaten
- 1 teaspoon tomato paste
- 1 tablespoon butter, melted
- Salt and pepper to taste
- 4 ounces French fries
- ¼ cup onions, diced
- 1 clove of garlic, minced
- ¾ cup cheddar cheese, grated

Instructions
1. In a mixing bowl, mix together the milk, eggs, tomato paste, and butter. Season with salt and pepper to taste. Set aside.
2. Place the French fries in the bottom of the Instant Pot.
3. Add the onions and garlic.
4. Pour the milk mixture and pour in the cheddar cheese.
5. Close the lid and seal off the vent.
6. Press the Manual button and add the adjust the cooking time to 10 minutes.
7. Do natural pressure release.

Nutrition information:
Calories per serving: 420; Carbohydrates: 26.3g; Protein: 24.7g; Fat: 24.3g; Fiber: 0.9g

Extra Thick Almond Milk Yogurt

Serves: 4
Preparation Time: 10 minutes
Cooking Time: 8 hours

Ingredients
- 4 cups almond milk
- 1/3 cup raw cashews
- 2 tablespoons arrowroot powder
- ¼ cup yogurt (source of live culture)
- 1 tablespoon maple syrup

Instructions
1. Place the almond milk, cashews and arrowroot powder in a blender. Pulse until smooth.
2. Transfer to a saucepan and heat over a medium flame while stirring constantly until the mixture simmers. Allow simmering for 5 minutes.
3. Remove from the heat to cool.
4. Transfer to the Instant Pot and add the yogurt with live culture.
5. Close the lid and press the Yogurt button. Adjust the cooking time to 8 hours.
6. Once the timer beeps, place the yogurt in clean mason jars and refrigerate before serving.
7. When ready to serve, drizzle with maple syrup or your favorite fruits.

Nutrition information:
Calories per serving: 285; Carbohydrates: 36.5g; Protein: 4.6g; Fat: 14.7g; Fiber: 1.7g

Blueberry Breakfast Oats

Serves: 1
Preparation Time: 3 minutes
Cooking Time: 6 minutes

Ingredients
- 1/3 cup old-fashioned oats
- 1/3 cup almond milk, unsweetened
- 1/3 cup Greek yogurt
- 1/3 cup blueberries
- 1 tablespoon chia seeds
- 2 tablespoons brown sugar
- A dash of salt
- A dash of cinnamon

Instructions
1. Place all ingredients in the Instant Pot and give a good stir.
2. Close the lid and seal the vent.
3. Press the Manual button and adjust the cooking time to 6 minutes.
4. Do natural pressure release.
5. Give a good stir before serving.

Nutrition information:
Calories per serving:343; Carbohydrates: 66.8g; Protein: 19.3g; Fat: 6.9g; Fiber: 9.9g

Instant Pot Banana Bread

Serves: 4
Preparation Time: 10 minutes
Cooking Time: 50 minutes

Ingredients
- 2 eggs, beaten
- 1 stick soft butter
- ½ cup sugar
- 4 bananas, mashed
- 1 tablespoon vanilla extract
- 2 cups flour
- 1 teaspoon baking powder

Instructions
1. Place a steamer rack in the Instant Pot and pour a cup of water into the pot.
2. In a mixing bowl, combine the eggs, butter, and sugar until creamy. Add the vanilla and bananas. Stir to mix well.
3. In another bowl, mix the flour and baking powder.
4. Gradually add the dry ingredients to the wet ingredients. Fold to combine everything.
5. Pour the batter into a greased baking dish that will fit inside the Instant Pot. Put foil over the top.
6. Place the baking dish on the steamer rack.
7. Close the lid and seal off the vent.
8. Press the Manual button and adjust the cooking time to 50 minutes.
9. Do quick pressure release and allow the banana bread to cool before serving.

Nutrition information:
Calories per serving: 554; Carbohydrates: 105.8g; Protein: 13.3g; Fat: 29.6g; Fiber: 6.7g

Egg and Broccoli Casserole

Serves: 6
Preparation Time: 5 minutes
Cooking Time: 15 minutes

Ingredients
- 3 cups cottage cheese
- 6 eggs, beaten
- 1/3 cup all-purpose flour
- ¼ cup butter, melted
- Salt and pepper to taste
- 3 cups broccoli florets
- 2 tablespoons chopped onions
- 2 cups cheddar cheese, grated

Instructions
1. In a mixing bowl, mix together the cottage cheese, eggs, all-purpose flour, butter, salt, and pepper. Mix until well-combined.
2. Place the broccoli and onions in the Instant Pot.
3. Pour over the egg mixture and sprinkle with grated cheese on top.
4. Close the lid and press the Manual button. Adjust the cooking time to 15 minutes.
5. Do natural pressure release.

Nutrition information:
Calories per serving:407; Carbohydrates: 15.8g; Protein: 27.8g; Fat: 25.7g; Fiber: 0.9g

Blueberry French Toast

Serves: 10
Preparation Time: 8 minutes
Cooking Time: 10 minutes

Ingredients
- 8 large eggs, lightly beaten
- ½ cup yogurt
- 1/3 cup sour cream
- 1 teaspoon vanilla extract
- ½ teaspoon ground cinnamon
- 1 cup milk
- 1-pound French bread, cubed
- 1 ½ cup blueberries
- 12 ounces cream cheese, cubed
- 1/3 cup maple syrup

Instructions
1. In a mixing bowl, combine the eggs, yogurt, sour cream, vanilla, cinnamon, and milk until well-combined.
2. Grease the inner pot of the Instant Pot with cooking spray.
3. Arrange the French bread, blueberries, and cream cheese in the Instant Pot.
4. Pour over the egg mixture and drizzle with maple syrup.
5. Close the lid and seal off the vent.
6. Press the Manual button and adjust the cooking time to 10 minutes.
7. Do natural pressure release.

Nutrition information:
Calories per serving: 363; Carbohydrates: 43.1g; Protein: 15g; Fat: 19g; Fiber:1.7 g

Delicious Egg Recipes

Instant Pot Egg Cups

Serves: 4
Preparation Time: 5 minutes
Cooking Time: 10 minutes
Ingredients
- 4 eggs
- 1 cup chopped frozen vegetables of your choice
- ½ cup cheddar cheese
- ¼ cup half and half
- Salt and pepper to taste

Instructions
1. Place a trivet or steamer basket inside the Instant Pot and pour water over.
2. In a mixing bowl, mix all ingredients until well combined.
3. Pour over greased ramekins until ¾ full.
4. Place aluminum foil over ramekins.
5. Place on the trivet.
6. Close the lid and seal off the vent.
7. Press the Manual button and adjust the cooking time to 10 minutes.
8. Do natural pressure release.

Nutrition information:
Calories per serving: 115; Carbohydrates: 2g; Protein: 9g; Fat: 9g; Fiber: 1.3g

Instant Pot Egg Muffins

Serves: 4
Preparation Time: 5 minutes
Cooking Time: 10 minutes
Ingredients
- 4 eggs
- ¼ teaspoon lemon pepper seasoning
- 4 tablespoons cheddar cheese, grated
- 1 green onion, diced
- 4 slices pre-cooked bacon, crumbled

Instructions
1. Place a trivet or steamer basket inside the Instant Pot and pour water over.
2. In a mixing bowl, mix all ingredients until well combined.
3. Pour over greased individual muffin cups until ¾ full.
4. Place aluminum foil over the muffin cups.
5. Place on the steamer basket.
6. Close the lid and seal off the vent.
7. Press the Manual button and adjust the cooking time to 10 minutes.
8. Do natural pressure release.

Nutrition information:
Calories per serving:484; Carbohydrates: 16.5g; Protein: 31.2g; Fat: 32.1g; Fiber: 0g

Instant Pot Breakfast Frittatas

Serves: 6
Preparation Time: 5 minutes
Cooking Time: 6 minutes
Ingredients
- 5 eggs
- ½ cup milk
- Salt and pepper to taste
- ¼ cup cheddar cheese
- ¼ cup ham, cubed

Instructions
1. In a mixing bowl, mix all ingredients until well combined.
2. Grease the inner pot of the Instant Pot.
3. Pour over the egg mixture.
4. Close the lid and press the Manual button.
5. Adjust the cooking time to 7 minutes.
6. Do natural pressure release.

Nutrition information:
Calories per serving: 242; Carbohydrates: 5.8g; Protein: 24.2g; Fat: 13.4g; Fiber: 0.1g

Basic Instant Pot Egg Salad Recipe

Serves: 12
Preparation Time: 5 minutes
Cooking Time: 10 minutes
Ingredients
- 12 eggs
- ½ cup mayonnaise
- Salt and pepper to taste

Instructions
1. Place a trivet or steamer basket inside the Instant Pot and pour water over.
2. In a mixing bowl, mix all ingredients until well combined.
3. Grease a baking dish that will fit in the Instant Pot.
4. Crack eggs into the baking dish. Place aluminum foil on top of the baking dish.
5. Close the lid and press the Manual button.
6. Adjust the cooking time to 10 minutes.
7. Do natural pressure release.
8. Mash the eggs with a fork and add in the mayonnaise. Season with salt and pepper to taste.

Nutrition information:
Calories per serving: 163; Carbohydrates: 1.7g; Protein: 9.6g; Fat: 12.8g; Fiber: 0.2g

Instant Pot Perfectly Soft-Boiled Eggs

Serves: 4
Preparation Time: 2 minutes
Cooking Time: 3 minutes
Ingredients
- 4 large eggs
- 1 cup water

Instructions
1. Place a trivet or steamer basket inside the Instant Pot and pour water over.
2. Place the eggs on top of the trivet.
3. Close the lid and press the Manual button.
4. Adjust the cooking time to 3 minutes.
5. Do quick pressure release.
6. Place the eggs in cold water to arrest the cooking process.

Nutrition information:
Calories per serving: 78; Carbohydrates: 0g; Protein: 6g; Fat: 5g; Fiber: 0g

Sous Vide Egg Bites

Serves: 4
Preparation Time: 5 minutes

Cooking Time: 15 minutes
Ingredients
- 4 large eggs, lightly beaten
- 4 cooked bacon strips, crumbled
- 1 ½ cups cheddar cheese, grated
- ½ cup cottage cheese
- ¼ cup heavy cream
- Salt and pepper to taste
- A dash of hot sauce

Instructions
1. Place a trivet or steamer basket inside the Instant Pot and pour water over.
2. Place bacon in small ramekins.
3. Place in the blender the eggs, cheese, cottage cheese, and cream. Season with salt and pepper to taste. Pulse until well-combined.
4. Pour into the ramekins until ¾ full. Cover with aluminum foil.
5. Close the lid and press the Manual button.
6. Adjust the cooking time to 15 minutes.
7. Do quick pressure release.
8. Drizzle with a dash of hot sauce.

Nutrition information:
Calories per serving: 375; Carbohydrates: 18.3g; Protein: 25.5g; Fat: 22.5g; Fiber: 0.3g

Instant Pot Scrambled Eggs

Serves: 2
Preparation Time: 2 minutes
Cooking Time: 3 minutes
Ingredients
- 2 eggs
- 1 tablespoon milk
- Salt and pepper to taste
- ½ tablespoon butter

Instructions
1. Place a trivet or steamer basket inside the Instant Pot and pour water over.
2. In a mixing bowl, combine the eggs and milk. Season with salt and pepper to taste.
3. Place the egg mixture into a heat-proof bowl that will fit in the Instant Pot.
4. Place the bowl with the egg mixture on the steamer basket.
5. Close the lid.
6. Press the Manual button and adjust the cooking time to 3 minutes.
7. Do natural pressure release.
8. Once the lid is open, add the butter and use a fork to fluff the eggs until they look like they are scrambled.

Nutrition information:
Calories per serving: 169; Carbohydrates: 3.5g; Protein: 9.7g; Fat: 12.8g; Fiber: 0.3g

Instant Pot Egg Custard

Serves: 6
Preparation Time: 5 minutes
Cooking Time: 10 minutes
Ingredients
- 4 cups of milk
- 6 large eggs, beaten
- ¾ cup white sugar
- 1 teaspoon vanilla extract
- A pinch of salt
- ¼ teaspoon ground cinnamon

Instructions
1. Place a trivet or steamer basket inside the Instant Pot and pour water over.
2. In a mixing bowl, combine all ingredients. Whisk until well-combined.
3. Place the egg mixture into a baking dish that will fit inside the Instant Pot. Cover with aluminum foil.
4. Place the baking dish with the egg mixture on the steamer basket.
5. Close the lid.
6. Press the Manual button and adjust the cooking time to 10 minutes.
7. Do natural pressure release.

Nutrition information:
Calories per serving:212; Carbohydrates: 11.7g; Protein:8.6 g; Fat: 14.6g; Fiber: 0.7g

Instant Pot Eggs in Marinara Sauce

Serves: 6
Preparation Time: 5 minutes
Cooking Time: 10 minutes
Ingredients
- 1 tablespoon coconut oil
- 2 cloves of garlic, minced
- ½ onion, diced
- 1 red bell pepper, diced
- 1 teaspoon chili powder
- ½ teaspoon paprika
- ½ teaspoon ground cumin
- Salt and pepper to taste
- 1 ½ cups commercial marinara sauce
- 6 eggs
- Parsley leaves for garnish

Instructions
1. Press the Sauté button on the Instant Pot.
2. Sauté the garlic and onions until fragrant.
3. Add the bell pepper, chili powder, paprika, and cumin. Season with salt and pepper to taste.
4. Continue stirring for 3 minutes.
5. Pour in the marinara sauce.
6. Gently crack the eggs into the marinara sauce.
7. Close the lid.
8. Press the Manual button and adjust the cooking time to 10 minutes.
9. Do natural pressure release.
10. Once the lid is opened, garnish with parsley.

Nutrition information:
Calories per serving: 182; Carbohydrates:8.4 g; Protein: 10.6g; Fat: 12.2g; Fiber: 1.8g

Indian Scrambled Eggs

Serves: 4
Preparation Time: 5 minutes
Cooking Time:3 minutes
Ingredients
- 6 eggs
- ¼ cup milk
- 1 tablespoon cooking oil
- 1 tablespoon ghee
- 1 large onion, chopped

- 2 cloves of garlic, minced
- 1 tomato, chopped
- 1 jalapeno pepper, chopped
- ½ inch ginger, grated
- 3 scallions, chopped
- ¼ teaspoon ground turmeric
- 1 teaspoon garam masala

Instructions
1. In a mixing bowl, combine the eggs and milk. Set aside.
2. Press the Sauté button on the Instant Pot.
3. Heat the oil and ghee.
4. Sauté the onion and garlic until fragrant.
5. Add the tomatoes, pepper, ginger, scallions, turmeric and garam masala. Continue stirring for 3 minutes.
6. Add the egg mixture.
7. Give a good stir.
8. Close the lid.
9. Press the Manual button and adjust the cooking time to 3 minutes.
10. Do natural pressure release.
11. Once the lid is open, fluff the eggs using two forks.

Nutrition information:
Calories per serving: 162; Carbohydrates: 8.3g; Protein: 9.7g; Fat: 10.3g; Fiber: 4.2g

Eggs and Chorizo

Serves: 3
Preparation Time: 5 minutes
Cooking Time: 10 minutes

Ingredients
- 1 tablespoon olive oil
- 1/3 cup onions, chopped
- ¼ pounds Mexican chorizo sausage, chopped
- 3 tablespoon raisins, soaked in water then drained
- 6 eggs
- Salt and pepper to taste

Instructions
1. Press the Sauté button on the Instant Pot.
2. Heat the oil and sauté the onions until fragrant.
3. Add in the chorizo sausages and continue stirring for 3 minutes.
4. Stir in the raisins and eggs.
5. Season with salt and pepper to taste.
6. Close the lid and press the Manual button.
7. Adjust the cooking time to 10 minutes.
8. Do natural pressure release.

Nutrition information:
Calories per serving: 409; Carbohydrates: 8.8g; Protein: 25.4g; Fat: 30.7g; Fiber: 1.5g

Asian Scrambled Eggs

Serves: 2
Preparation Time: 5 minutes
Cooking Time: 15 minutes

Ingredients
- 4 large eggs, beaten
- 1 tablespoon light soy sauce
- ½ teaspoon oyster sauce
- 2 tomatoes, sliced
- 1 tablespoon oil
- ½ cup chicken stock
- 1 tablespoon potato starch

Instructions
1. In a mixing bowl, mix all ingredients until well combined.
2. Pour over the Instant Pot.
3. Close the lid and press the Manual button.
4. Adjust the cooking time to 15 minutes.
5. Do natural pressure release.
6. Once the lid is open, fluff the eggs using a fork.

Nutrition information:
Calories per serving: 278; Carbohydrates: 13.4g; Protein: 15.6g; Fat: 17.2g; Fiber: 1.8g

Instant Pot Poblano Cheese Frittata

Serves: 4
Preparation Time: 5 minutes
Cooking Time: 10 minutes

Ingredients
- 4 eggs
- 1 cup half and half
- ½ teaspoon salt
- ½ teaspoon cumin
- 10 ounces canned green chilies, chopped
- 1 cup Mexican cheese blend, grated
- ½ cup cilantro, chopped

Instructions
1. Place a trivet or steamer basket inside the Instant Pot and pour water over.
2. In a mixing bowl, combine the eggs and half-and-half. Season with salt and cumin. Whisk until well-combined.
3. Place the egg mixture into a baking dish that will fit inside the Instant Pot.
4. Add the chilies and top with Mexican cheese blend.
5. Cover the baking dish with aluminum foil.
6. Place the baking dish with the egg mixture on the steamer basket.
7. Close the lid.
8. Press the Manual button and adjust the cooking time to 10 minutes.
9. Do natural pressure release.
10. Garnish with chopped cilantro.

Nutrition information:
Calories per serving: 257; Carbohydrates: 6g; Protein: 14.2g; Fat:19g; Fiber: 1.5g

Herbed Crustless Quiche

Serves: 8
Preparation Time: 5 minutes
Cooking Time: 15 minutes

Ingredients
- 4 eggs
- 1 cup milk
- 1/3 cup flour
- ¼ teaspoon baking soda
- ½ teaspoon salt
- ½ teaspoon thyme
- 1 tablespoon parsley
- 1/8 teaspoon paprika
- A dash of crushed red pepper
- ½ teaspoon dill
- Salt and pepper to taste
- 1 cup spinach, chopped

- 2 scallions, chopped
- ½ cup broccoli, chopped
- ½ red bell pepper, chopped
- ½ cup goat cheese, cubed

Instructions
1. Place a trivet or steamer basket inside the Instant Pot and pour water over.
2. In a mixing bowl, combine the eggs, milk, flour, baking soda, salt, thyme, parsley, paprika, crushed red pepper, and dill. Season with salt and pepper to taste.
3. Place the egg mixture into a baking dish that will fit inside the Instant Pot.
4. Stir in the spinach, scallions, broccoli, red bell pepper, and goat cheese.
5. Cover the baking dish with aluminum foil.
6. Place the baking dish with the egg mixture on the steamer basket.
7. Close the lid.
8. Press the Manual button and adjust the cooking time to 15 minutes.
9. Do natural pressure release.

Nutrition information:
Calories per serving: 122; Carbohydrates: 7.9g; Protein: 7.3g; Fat: 6.8g; Fiber: 0.7g

Asparagus and Chive Frittata

Serves: 6
Preparation Time: 5 minutes
Cooking Time: 10 minutes

Ingredients
- 6 large eggs
- ½ cup milk
- ¼ teaspoon salt
- A pinch of black pepper
- 1 cup cheddar cheese, grated
- 2 tablespoons chives, chopped
- 1 cup asparagus heads, trimmed

Instructions
1. Place a trivet or steamer basket inside the Instant Pot and pour water over.
2. In a mixing bowl, combine the eggs and milk. Season with salt and pepper.
3. Place the egg mixture into a baking dish that will fit inside the Instant Pot.
4. Stir in the cheddar cheese, chives, and asparagus heads.
5. Cover the baking dish with aluminum foil.
6. Place the baking dish with the egg mixture on the steamer basket.
7. Close the lid.
8. Press the Manual button and adjust the cooking time to 10 minutes.
9. Do natural pressure release.

Nutrition information:
Calories per serving: 103; Carbohydrates: 7.6g; Protein: 8.4g; Fat: 4.9g; Fiber: 0.6g

Sausage, Ham, And Cheese Quiche

Serves: 5
Preparation Time: 6 minutes
Cooking Time: 10 minutes

Ingredients
- 1 baking potatoes, sliced thinly
- 2 links of chicken sausages, sliced
- ½ cup ham, chopped
- 3 eggs
- 1 cup milk
- Salt and pepper to taste
- 1 cup cheddar cheese, grated

Instructions
1. Place a trivet or steamer basket inside the Instant Pot and pour water over.
2. Grease a baking pan that will fit inside the Instant Pot with cooking spray.
3. Layer the baking potatoes at the bottom followed by the chicken sausages and ham.
4. In a mixing bowl, combine the eggs and milk. Season with salt and pepper to taste.
5. Place the egg mixture into a baking dish with the potatoes, chicken, and ham.
6. Sprinkle with grated cheese on top.
7. Cover the baking dish with aluminum foil.
8. Place the baking dish with the egg mixture on the steamer basket.
9. Close the lid.
10. Press the Manual button and adjust the cooking time to 10 minutes.
11. Do natural pressure release.

Nutrition information:
Calories per serving: 282; Carbohydrates: 18.9g; Protein: 24.1g; Fat: 11.9g; Fiber: 1.2g

Bacon and Broccoli Quiche

Serves: 6
Preparation Time: 5 minutes
Cooking Time: 15 minutes

Ingredients
- 6 eggs
- 2 teaspoon dry mustard
- ½ cup milk
- ¼ teaspoon salt
- A pinch of ground black pepper
- 1 cup cheddar cheese, grated
- 8 slices of bacon, cooked and crumbled
- 2 tablespoons green onions, chopped

Instructions
1. Place a trivet or steamer basket inside the Instant Pot and pour water over.
2. In a mixing bowl, combine the eggs, mustard, and milk. Season with salt and pepper to taste.
3. Place the egg mixture into a baking dish that will fit inside the Instant Pot.
4. Sprinkle with grated cheese on top.
5. Cover the baking dish with aluminum foil.
6. Place the baking dish with the egg mixture on the steamer basket.
7. Close the lid.
8. Press the Manual button and adjust the cooking time to 15 minutes.
9. Do natural pressure release.
10. Once the lid is open, sprinkle with bacon and green onions.

Nutrition information:
Calories per serving: 317; Carbohydrates: 4.9g; Protein: 16.4g; Fat: 25.4g; Fiber: 0.2g

Instant Pot Southwest Biscuit Egg Bake

Serves: 5
Preparation Time: 10 minutes
Cooking Time: 15 minutes
Ingredients
- 3 buttermilk biscuits
- 6 eggs
- ½ cup milk
- 2 tablespoons chives
- ½ cup salsa
- 1 tablespoon green chilies, chopped
- ¼ teaspoon garlic powder
- ¼ teaspoon dried oregano
- Salt and pepper to taste
- 1 cup cheddar cheese, grated

Instructions
1. Place a trivet or steamer basket inside the Instant Pot and pour water over.
2. Line a baking dish that will fit inside the Instant Pot with buttermilk biscuits. Set aside.
3. In a mixing bowl, combine the eggs, milk, chives, salsa, green chilies, garlic powder, and dried oregano. Season with salt and pepper to taste.
4. Place the egg mixture into a baking dish that will fit inside the Instant Pot.
5. Sprinkle with grated cheese on top.
6. Cover the baking dish with aluminum foil.
7. Place the baking dish with the egg mixture on the steamer basket.
8. Close the lid.
9. Press the Manual button and adjust the cooking time to 15 minutes.
10. Do natural pressure release.

Nutrition information:
Calories per serving:317; Carbohydrates: 22.4g; Protein: 16.9g; Fat: 17.7g; Fiber: 1.6g

Easy Instant Pot Poached Eggs

Serves: 5
Preparation Time: 5 minutes
Cooking Time: 5 minutes
Ingredients
- 5 eggs
- 1 cup water

Instructions
1. Place a trivet or steamer basket inside the Instant Pot and pour water over.
2. Spray 5 silicone cups with cooking spray.
3. Crack each egg into each greased cup.
4. Place the silicone cups with eggs on the steamer.
5. Close the lid.
6. Press the Steam button and adjust the cooking time to 5 minutes.
7. Do quick pressure release.

Nutrition information:
Calories per serving:130; Carbohydrates: 1.1g; Protein: 8.7g; Fat: 9.6g; Fiber: 0g

Instant Pot Hong Kong Egg Custard

Serves: 5
Preparation Time: 15 minutes
Cooking Time: 8 minutes
Ingredients
- 1 ½ cups whole milk warm
- 5 tablespoons granulated sugar
- 1 pinch of salt
- 3 eggs

Instructions
1. Place a trivet or steamer basket inside the Instant Pot and pour water over.
2. In a mixing bowl, combine the warm milk and sugar. Add the salt. Mix until the sugar granules have melted.
3. Pass through a sieve to remove any lumps.
4. In a separate glass bowl, beat the eggs until well blended.
5. Slowly pour the milk mixture into the eggs while beating constantly.
6. Strain the egg mixture and place into a baking dish or smaller ramekins that will fit inside the Instant Pot.
7. Cover the dish with aluminum foil.
8. Place the dish with the egg mixture on the steamer basket.
9. Close the lid.
10. Press the Manual button and adjust the cooking time to 8 minutes.
11. Do natural pressure release.

Nutrition information:
Calories per serving:119; Carbohydrates: 13g; Protein: 5g; Fat: 4g; Fiber: 0g

Cheesy Egg Casserole

Serves: 12
Preparation Time: 5 minutes
Cooking Time:15 minutes
Ingredients
- ½ cup butter, melted
- 1 package cottage cheese
- ¼ cup all-purpose flour
- 1 teaspoon baking powder
- 1 teaspoon Italian seasoning
- ½ teaspoon salt
- 10 eggs, lightly beaten
- 2 cups mozzarella cheese, grated

Instructions
1. Place a trivet or steamer basket inside the Instant Pot and pour water over.
2. In a mixing bowl, combine all ingredients except the mozzarella cheese. Stir until well combined.
3. Place the egg mixture into a baking dish that will fit inside the Instant Pot.
4. Sprinkle with grated mozzarella cheese on top.
5. Cover the baking dish with aluminum foil.
6. Place the baking dish with the egg mixture on the steamer basket.
7. Close the lid.
8. Press the Manual button and adjust the cooking time to 15 minutes.
9. Do natural pressure release.

Nutrition information:
Calories per serving: 238; Carbohydrates: 4.4g; Protein: 15.6g; Fat: 17.5g; Fiber: 0.5g

Instant Pot Deviled Eggs

Serves: 16
Preparation Time: 15 minutes

Cooking Time: 12 minutes
Ingredients
- 8 large eggs
- 1 cup cold water
- 2 tablespoons full-fat mayonnaise
- 1 tablespoon olive oil
- 1 teaspoon Dijon mustard
- 1 teaspoon white vinegar
- ¼ teaspoon sriracha
- Salt and pepper to taste

Instructions
1. Place a trivet or steamer basket inside the Instant Pot and pour water the water inside.
2. Place the eggs in the steamer basket.
3. Close the lid and press the Steam button. Set the pressure to Low and adjust the cooking time to 12 minutes.
4. Do quick pressure release.
5. Once the eggs are out, submerge in cold water for 5 minutes.
6. Crack open the egg shells.
7. Slice the eggs lengthwise and remove the yolks. Place the yolks in a bowl and add in the rest of the ingredients.
8. Place the yolk mixture into piping bags and pipe carefully back into the depression within the egg whites.

Nutrition information:
Calories per serving:39; Carbohydrates: 0.8g; Protein: 1.6g; Fat:3.3g; Fiber: 0.1g

Instant Pot Lemon Orzo Soup

Serves: 4
Preparation Time: 5 minutes
Cooking Time: 10 minutes
Ingredients
- 6 cups chicken broth
- ¾ cup uncooked orzo or small pasta
- 3 eggs
- Juice of 2 lemons, freshly squeezed

Instructions
1. Place the broth and orzo into the Instant Pot.
2. Close the lid and press the Manual button.
3. Adjust the cooking time to 5 minutes.
4. Do quick pressure release.
5. Once the lid is removed, press the Sauté button and stir in the eggs and lemon juice.
6. Stir lightly.

Nutrition information:
Calories per serving: 704; Carbohydrates: 12.5g; Protein: 85.3g; Fat:32.5g; Fiber: 1.3g

Instant Pot Hard Boiled Egg Loaf

Serves: 3
Preparation Time: 5 minutes
Cooking Time: 6 minutes
Ingredients
- Cooking spray
- 6 eggs

Instructions
1. Grease the loaf pan that will fit inside the Instant Pot.
2. Crack the eggs carefully into the greased pot.
3. Place a trivet or steamer basket inside the Instant Pot and pour water the water inside.
4. Place the loaf pan with the eggs on top of the steamer.
5. Close the lid and press the Manual button.
6. Adjust the cooking time to 6 minutes.
7. Do quick pressure release.

Nutrition information:
Calories per serving: 259; Carbohydrates:2.1 g; Protein: 17.9g; Fat: 19.3g; Fiber: 0g

Instant Pot Bacon and Broccoli Frittata

Serves: 6
Preparation Time: 10 minutes
Cooking Time: 20 minutes
Ingredients
- 4 eggs
- ¼ cup milk
- 1 teaspoon salt
- Zest of 1 lemon
- 1 tablespoon Italian parsley, chopped
- 1 teaspoon fresh thyme
- Salt and pepper
- 2 tablespoons butter, melted
- 1 onion, diced
- 4 cloves of garlic, grated
- 1 cup broccoli florets
- 1 ½ cups cheddar cheese, grated
- 8 slices turkey bacon, fried and crumbled

Instructions
1. In a mixing bowl, combine the eggs, milk, salt, lemon zest, parsley, and thyme. Season with salt and pepper to taste. Set aside.
2. Press the Sauté button in the Instant Pot.
3. Heat the butter and sauté the onion and garlic.
4. Add the broccoli florets.
5. Pour in the eggs mixture and sprinkle with cheese on top.
6. Close the lid and press the Manual button.
7. Adjust the cooking time to 15 minutes.
8. Do quick pressure release.
9. Sprinkle with turkey bacon bits.

Nutrition information:
Calories per serving: 298; Carbohydrates: 10.4g; Protein: 18.6g; Fat: 20.3g; Fiber: 0.7g

Turkey Egg Breakfast Casserole

Serves: 12
Preparation Time: 5 minutes
Cooking Time: 10 minutes
Ingredients
- 1 tablespoon coconut oil
- 1-pound ground turkey
- ½ teaspoon chili powder
- Salt and pepper to taste
- 1 cup baby spinach, chopped
- 12 large eggs, beaten

Instructions
1. Press the Sauté button on the Instant Pot.
2. Heat the coconut oil and add on the ground turkey.
3. Stir and cook for 3 minutes until the turkey has browned. Add the chili powder and season with salt and pepper to taste.

4. Stir in the spinach and pour over the beaten eggs.
5. Close the lid and press the Manual button.
6. Adjust the cooking time to 10 minutes.
7. Do natural pressure release.
Nutrition information:
Calories per serving: 276; Carbohydrates: 5g; Protein:20g; Fat: 18g; Fiber:1 g

Simple Egg Casserole
Serves: 8
Preparation Time: 5 minutes
Cooking Time: 15 minutes
Ingredients
- 1 package sausage, chopped
- 8 eggs, beaten
- 1 cup milk
- Salt and pepper to taste
- 1 cup mozzarella cheese, shredded

Instructions
1. Place a trivet or steamer basket inside the Instant Pot and pour water over.
2. In a mixing bowl, combine all ingredients except the mozzarella cheese. Stir until well combined.
3. Place the egg mixture into a baking dish that will fit inside the Instant Pot.
4. Sprinkle with grated mozzarella cheese on top.
5. Cover the baking dish with aluminum foil.
6. Place the baking dish with the egg mixture on the steamer basket.
7. Close the lid.
8. Press the Manual button and adjust the cooking time to 15 minutes.
9. Do natural pressure release.
Nutrition information:
Calories per serving: 251; Carbohydrates:6.6 g; Protein: 20.3g; Fat: 16.3g; Fiber: 1.2g

Potato Bacon Egg Breakfast
Serves: 6
Preparation Time: 5 minutes
Cooking Time: 15 minutes
Ingredients
- 8 large eggs
- ½ cup whole milk
- 2 small potatoes, peeled and chopped
- Salt and pepper to taste
- 10 pieces of bacon, fried and crumbled

Instructions
1. Place a trivet or steamer basket inside the Instant Pot and pour water over.
2. In a mixing bowl, combine all ingredients except the bacon bits. Stir until well combined.
3. Place the egg mixture into a baking dish that will fit inside the Instant Pot.
4. Cover the baking dish with aluminum foil.
5. Place the baking dish with the egg mixture on the steamer basket.
6. Close the lid.
7. Press the Manual button and adjust the cooking time to 15 minutes.
8. Do natural pressure release.
9. Sprinkle with bacon bits on top.
Nutrition information:
Calories per serving: 215; Carbohydrates: 26.2g; Protein:7.7 g; Fat: 9.3g; Fiber: 3g

Sausages and Eggs
Serves: 8
Preparation Time: 5 minutes
Cooking Time: 20 minutes
Ingredients
- 1 loaf Italian bread, sliced
- 1-pound breakfast sausage, chopped
- 1 cup cheddar cheese, grated
- 8 eggs
- 1 cup milk
- Salt and pepper
- 1 cup mozzarella cheese, grated

Instructions
1. Place a trivet or steamer basket inside the Instant Pot and pour water over.
2. Grease a baking dish that will fit in the Instant Pot.
3. Arrange the Italian bread slices at the bottom.
4. Add the sausages and cheddar cheese for the next layers.
5. In a mixing bowl, combine the eggs and milk. Season with salt and pepper. Stir until well combined.
6. Pour over the egg mixture into the dish with the layers of ingredients.
7. Sprinkle with mozzarella cheese on top.
8. Cover the baking dish with aluminum foil.
9. Place the baking dish with the egg mixture on the steamer basket.
10. Close the lid.
11. Press the Steam button and adjust the cooking time to 20 minutes.
12. Do natural pressure release.
Nutrition information:
Calories per serving:547; Carbohydrates: 23.9g; Protein: 28.2g; Fat: 37g; Fiber: 1.1g

5-Ingredient Shakshuka
Serves: 4
Preparation Time: 5 minutes
Cooking Time: 15 minutes
Ingredients
- 1 onion, sliced
- 1 ½ cups sweet bell pepper, pureed
- 2 cans diced tomatoes
- 2 tablespoons red pepper flakes
- Salt and pepper
- 4 eggs
- ½ cup flat-leaf parsley

Instructions
1. Place the onions, sweet bell pepper puree, diced tomatoes, and red pepper flakes in the Instant Pot.
2. Season with salt and pepper to taste. Give a stir to combine everything.
3. Carefully crack the eggs into the Instant Pot.
4. Sprinkle with half of the parsley.
5. Close the lid.
6. Press the Manual button and adjust the cooking time to 15 minutes.
7. Do natural pressure release.
8. Sprinkle with the remaining parsley.
Nutrition information:

Calories per serving:241; Carbohydrates:11 g; Protein: 10g; Fat:5 g; Fiber: 6g

Pepperoni and Potato Frittata

Serves: 12
Preparation Time: 10 minutes
Cooking Time: 20 minutes
Ingredients
- 3 medium-sized potatoes, unpeeled and sliced
- ½ of pepperoni salami, sliced
- 1 onion, sliced
- 10 eggs
- ¼ cup milk
- Salt and pepper to taste
- 1 ½ tablespoons fresh thyme leaves
- ½ cup cheddar cheese

Instructions
1. Place a trivet or steamer basket inside the Instant Pot and pour water over.
2. Grease a baking dish that will fit in the Instant Pot.
3. Arrange the potatoes and salami at the bottom of the baking dish. Add the onions.
4. In a mixing bowl, combine the eggs and milk. Season with salt and pepper to taste. Add the thyme.
5. Pour the egg mixture into the baking dish with the potatoes and salami.
6. Cover the baking dish with aluminum foil.
7. Place the baking dish with the egg mixture on the steamer basket.
8. Close the lid.
9. Press the Steam button and adjust the cooking time to 20 minutes.
10. Do natural pressure release.

Nutrition information:
Calories per serving: 227; Carbohydrates: 21.1g; Protein: 11.7g; Fat: 10.6g; Fiber: 2.3 g

Zucchini and Eggs

Serves: 10
Preparation Time: 5 minutes
Cooking Time: 15 minutes
Ingredients
- 8 eggs
- ½ cups milk
- 3 tablespoons butter, melted
- 2 cloves of garlic, minced
- 1 onion, chopped
- 2 zucchinis, sliced
- 1 tablespoon fresh oregano
- Salt and pepper to taste
- 1 ½ cups cheddar cheese, grated

Instructions
1. In a mixing bowl, mix together the eggs and milk. Set aside.
2. Press the Sauté button on the Instant Pot. Heat the butter.
3. Sauté the garlic and onions until fragrant.
4. Add the zucchini slices and oregano. Season with salt and pepper to taste.
5. Pour in the egg mixture.
6. Sprinkle with cheese on top.
7. Close the lid.

8. Press the Manual button and adjust the cooking time to 15 minutes.
9. Do natural pressure release.

Nutrition information:
Calories per serving: 326; Carbohydrates: 10.5g; Protein: 18.3 g; Fat: 18.1g; Fiber: 2.2g

Silver Beet and Dukkah Baked Eggs

Serves: 4
Preparation Time: 5 minutes
Cooking Time: 10 minutes
Ingredients
- 1 tablespoon olive oil
- 1 onion, chopped
- 2 cloves of garlic, chopped
- 1 can diced tomatoes
- 1 cup red bell pepper, chopped
- 1 bunch silver beet, leaves chopped
- 4 eggs
- 1 cup feta cheese, crumbled
- ¼ cup mint leaves chopped
- 2 tablespoon lemon juice

Instructions
1. Press the Sauté button on the Instant Pot.
2. Heat the oil and sauté the onion and garlic until fragrant.
3. Stir in the tomatoes, red bell peppers, and silver beet leaves.
4. Continue stirring until the silver beet leaves have wilted.
5. Make 4 depressions in the mixture and, to each, crack open an egg.
6. Sprinkle with feta cheese and mint leaves on top.
7. Close the lid and press the Manual button.
8. Adjust the cooking time to 10 minutes.
9. Do natural pressure release.
10. Drizzle with lemon juice on top.
11. Serve with pita bread.

Nutrition information:
Calories per serving: 316; Carbohydrates: 14.3g; Protein: 21.5g; Fat: 21.6g; Fiber: 2.6g

Chives and Eggs Casserole

Serves: 8
Preparation Time: 5 minutes
Cooking Time: 15 minutes
Ingredients
- ½ cups chives, chopped
- 8 eggs
- ½ cups milk
- Salt and pepper to taste

Instructions
1. Place a trivet or steamer basket inside the Instant Pot and pour water over.
2. Grease a baking dish that will fit in the Instant Pot.
3. In a mixing bowl, combine all ingredients.
4. Pour the egg mixture into the baking dish.
5. Cover the baking dish with aluminum foil.
6. Place the baking dish with the egg mixture on the steamer basket.
7. Close the lid.
8. Press the Steam button and adjust the cooking time to 15 minutes.

9. Do natural pressure release.
Nutrition information:
Calories per serving: 142; Carbohydrates: 2.4g; Protein: 9.6g; Fat: 10.2g; Fiber: 0.1g

Spinach Baked Eggs with Parmesan on Toast

Serves: 4
Preparation Time: 5 minutes
Cooking Time: 15 minutes
Ingredients
- 1 cup spinach
- ½ cup parmesan
- 4 eggs
- Salt and pepper to taste
- 8 slices French stick bread, toasted

Instructions
1. Place a trivet or steamer basket inside the Instant Pot and pour water over.
2. Grease a baking dish that will fit in the Instant Pot.
3. In a mixing bowl, combine all ingredients except for the French stick bread.
4. Pour the egg mixture into the baking dish.
5. Cover the baking dish with aluminum foil.
6. Place the baking dish with the egg mixture on the steamer basket.
7. Close the lid.
8. Press the Steam button and adjust the cooking time to 15 minutes.
9. Do natural pressure release.
10. Serve with the bread.

Nutrition information:
Calories per serving: 530; Carbohydrates: 28.1g; Protein: 32.8g; Fat: 31.6g; Fiber: 0.5g

One-Pan Eggs and Peppers

Serves: 4
Preparation Time:
Cooking Time:
Ingredients
- 2 tablespoons olive oil
- 2 cloves of garlic
- 2 onions, chopped
- 1 red or green bell pepper, deseeded and sliced
- 2 red chilies, chopped
- 1 can crushed tomatoes
- 2 teaspoons caster sugar
- Salt and pepper
- 4 eggs, lightly beaten
- 1 bunch parsley, chopped
- 6 tablespoons creamy yogurt, for garnish

Instructions
1. Press the Sauté button on the Instant Pot and heat the oil.
2. Sauté the garlic and onions until fragrant.
3. Stir in the bell pepper, chilies, and tomatoes. Season with sugar, salt, and pepper.
4. Pour in the eggs and parsley.
5. Close the lid.
6. Press the Manual button and adjust the cooking time to 6 minutes.
7. Do natural pressure release.
8. Garnish with yogurt on top.

Nutrition information:
Calories per serving: 222; Carbohydrates: 12g; Protein 1.3 g; Fat:14 g; Fiber: 3g

Instant Pot Coddled Eggs

Serves: 4
Preparation Time: 5 minutes
Cooking Time: 10 minutes
Ingredients
- 3 tablespoons butter
- 1 onion, chopped
- ¼ cup white wine
- 1 cup chicken stock
- 1 cup heavy cream
- 1 cup arugula leaves
- 4 eggs, lightly beaten
- 4 bacon strips, fried and crumbled

Instructions
1. Press the Sauté button on the Instant Pot.
2. Heat the butter and sauté the onion until fragrant.
3. Add the white wine, chicken stock, and heavy cream.
4. Close the lid.
5. Press the Manual button and adjust the cooking time to 6 minutes.
6. Do quick natural release.
7. Once the lid is open, press the Sauté button and select the high setting.
8. Add the arugula leaves and eggs. Stir constantly until the mixture thickens.
9. Garnish with bacon strips.
10. Serve on toast.

Nutrition information:
Calories per serving: 360; Carbohydrates: 7.2g; Protein: 12.2g; Fat: 31.6g; Fiber: 2.5g

Baked Eggs with Chorizo

Serves: 8
Preparation Time: 5 minutes
Cooking Time:15 minutes
Ingredients
- 2 tablespoons olive oil
- 1 onion, diced
- 2 cloves of garlic, minced
- 1 tablespoon paprika
- 2 chorizo sausages, sliced
- 1 can diced tomatoes
- ½ cup frozen peas
- Salt and pepper
- 8 eggs, lightly beaten
- 1 cup mozzarella cheese, grated
- ¼ cup parsley, chopped

Instructions
1. Press the Sauté button on the Instant Pot.
2. Heat the oil and sauté the onion and garlic until fragrant.
3. Add the paprika and sausages.
4. Continue stirring for another 3 minutes.
5. Stir in the diced tomatoes including the liquid.
6. Add the peas and season with salt and pepper. Give a good stir.
7. Stir in the beaten eggs.
8. Sprinkle with cheese on top.

9. Close the lid.
10. Press the Manual button and adjust the cooking time to 15 minutes.
11. Do quick natural release.
12. Once open, garnish with parsley.
Nutrition information:
Calories per serving: 217; Carbohydrates: 6.3g; Protein: 15.6g; Fat: 14.5g; Fiber: 1.9g

Romesco Eggs with Sausages

Serves: 4
Preparation Time: 5 minutes
Cooking Time: 15 minutes
Ingredients
- 1 tablespoon oil
- 1 cup chopped sausages
- ½ cup chopped onions
- 2 cloves of garlic, minced
- 1 cup Romesco sauce
- 1 ½ cup tomato sauce
- 2 tomatoes, chopped
- Salt and pepper
- 4 eggs, lightly beaten

Instructions
1. Press the Sauté button on the Instant Pot.
2. Heat the oil and sauté the sausages together with the onion and garlic until fragrant.
3. Pour in the Romesco sauce, tomato sauce, and tomatoes. Season with salt and pepper to taste.
4. Add the beaten eggs.
5. Close the lid.
6. Press the Manual button and adjust the cooking time to 15 minutes.
7. Do quick natural release.

Nutrition information:
Calories per serving:469; Carbohydrates: 37.4g; Protein: 25.1g; Fat: 24.9g; Fiber: 10.2g

Egg Masala Curry

Serves: 6
Preparation Time: 5 minutes
Cooking Time: 10 minutes
Ingredients
- 6 eggs
- 2 tablespoons oil
- 1 onion, chopped
- ½ teaspoon turmeric powder
- ½ teaspoon chili powder
- 1 thumb-size ginger
- 1 green chili, sliced
- ½ teaspoon garam masala
- 1 can coconut milk
- ½ cup coriander leaves

Instructions
1. Place a trivet or steamer basket inside the Instant Pot and pour water over.
2. Arrange the eggs on the steamer basket.
3. Close the lid and press the Steam button. Adjust the cooking time to 6 minutes.
4. Do natural pressure release.
5. Peel the eggs and set aside.
6. Clean the inner pot and press the Sauté button.
7. Add the oil and sauté the onion, turmeric powder, chili powder, ginger, chili, and garam masala until fragrant.
8. Add coconut milk and eggs.
9. Close the lid.
10. Press the Manual button and adjust the cooking time to 3 minutes.
11. Do quick pressure release.
12. Garnish with coriander leaves.
13. Serve with rice.

Nutrition information:
Calories per serving: 352; Carbohydrates: 16g; Protein: 18.5g; Fat: 28.4g; Fiber: 4g

Eggs in Pots with Smoked Salmon Casserole

Serves: 8
Preparation Time: 5 minutes
Cooking Time: 15 minutes
Ingredients
- 2 tablespoons olive oil
- 2 leeks, sliced
- ½ cup peas
- 2 teaspoon lemon zest
- 2/3 cup cooking cream
- 1 cup smoked salmon flakes
- 1 tablespoon thyme
- Salt and pepper to taste
- 8 eggs, beaten

Instructions
1. Press the Sauté button on the Instant Pot.
2. Heat the oil and sauté the leeks until fragrant.
3. Add the peas and lemon zest.
4. Stir in the cooking cream and salmon flakes.
5. Season with thyme, salt, and pepper.
6. Pour in the beaten eggs.
7. Close the lid.
8. Press the Manual button and adjust the cooking time to 15 minutes.
9. Do quick natural release.

Nutrition information:
Calories per serving: 219; Carbohydrates: 8.1g; Protein: 13.5g; Fat: 14.5g; Fiber: 1.6g

Toad-in-the-hole Eggs and Tomatoes

Serves: 3
Preparation Time: 5 minutes
Cooking Time: 20 minutes
Ingredients
- 3 eggs
- 1 cup milk
- 1 tablespoon Dijon mustard
- 1 ½ tablespoons oil
- 8 sausages, chopped
- 1 tablespoon rosemary leaves
- 1 onion, sliced
- 1 cup green beans, sliced
- 1 can crushed tomatoes
- Salt and pepper to taste

Instructions
1. In a mixing bowl, combine the eggs and milk. Season with Dijon mustard. Set aside.

2. Press the Sauté button on the Instant Pot and add the sausages, rosemary leaves, and onions. Stir until fragrant.
3. Add the green beans and tomatoes. Season with salt and pepper. Stir until well combined.
4. Create a big depression in the middle and pour in the egg mixture.
5. Close the lid.
6. Press the Manual button and adjust the cooking time to 15 minutes.
7. Do quick natural release.

Nutrition information:
Calories per serving: 443; Carbohydrates: 17.7g; Protein: 25.5g; Fat: 31.8g; Fiber: 4.6g

Simple Savory Tomatoes and Eggs

Serves: 4
Preparation Time: 5 minutes
Cooking Time: 15 minutes

Ingredients
- 4 eggs, beaten
- 1 cup chicken stock
- 2 teaspoons olive oil
- 1 onion, chopped
- 2 cloves of garlic, minced
- 2 sausages, chopped
- ½ teaspoon smoked paprika
- A dash of chili flakes
- 1 can crushed tomatoes
- 3 teaspoons red wine vinegar
- Salt and pepper
- 1 cup parmesan cheese

Instructions
1. In a mixing bowl, mix together the eggs and chicken stock. Set aside.
2. Press the Sauté button on the Instant Pot and heat the oil.
3. Sauté the onion and garlic until fragrant.
4. Add in the sausages, paprika, and chili flakes. Continue stirring for 3 minutes.
5. Add the tomatoes and red wine. Season with salt and pepper to taste.
6. Pour in the egg mixture.
7. Close the lid.
8. Press the Manual button and adjust the cooking time to 15 minutes.
9. Do quick natural release.
10. Sprinkle with parmesan cheese on top.

Nutrition information:
Calories per serving: 335; Carbohydrates: 13.8g; Protein: 20.9g; Fat: 22.1g; Fiber: 2.1g

Chorizo, Kale and Apple Frittata

Serves: 9
Preparation Time: 5 minutes
Cooking Time: 15 minutes

Ingredients
- 9 eggs
- 1 cup milk
- 1 tablespoon olive oil
- 1 link classic chorizo, chopped
- 1 onion, sliced
- 1 red apple, cored and chopped
- 1 cup kale sliced

Instructions
1. In a mixing bowl, combine the eggs and milk. Set aside.
2. Press the Sauté button on the Instant Pot.
3. Heat the oil and sauté the chorizo and onions. Stir in the apples and kales.
4. Pour over the egg mixture.
5. Close the lid.
6. Press the Manual button and adjust the cooking time to 15 minutes.
7. Do quick natural release.

Nutrition information:
Calories per serving: 205; Carbohydrates: 6g; Protein: 11.6g; Fat: 14.8g; Fiber: 0.9g

Mexican Eggs with Potato Hash

Serves: 4
Preparation Time: 5 minutes
Cooking Time: 20 minutes

Ingredients
- 1 tablespoon oil
- 1 onion, chopped
- ½ pound ground beef
- Salt and pepper to taste
- ½ pounds potatoes, grated
- ¼ cup chipotle chili sauce
- 1 can tomatoes, chopped
- 1/3 cup coriander, chopped
- 4 eggs, beaten

Instructions
1. Press the Sauté button on the Instant Pot.
2. Sauté the onion and ground beef for three minutes until fragrant. Season with salt and pepper to taste. Set aside.
3. Turn off the Instant Pot.
4. Arrange the grated potatoes at the bottom of the Instant Pot.
5. Pour in the beef mixture, chipotle sauce, tomatoes, and coriander.
6. Pour over beaten eggs.
7. Close the lid.
8. Press the Manual button and adjust the cooking time to 15 minutes.
9. Do quick natural release.

Nutrition information:
Calories per serving: 388; Carbohydrates: 19.6g; Protein: 25.7g; Fat: 22.9g; Fiber: 3.8g

Beans Recipes

Pinto Beans with Chorizo

Serves: 6
Preparation Time: 5 minutes
Cooking Time: 40 minutes
Ingredients
- 1 tablespoon cooking oil
- 4 ounces chorizo, chopped
- 1 onion, chopped
- 3 cloves of garlic, minced
- 2 cups dry pinto beans, soaked overnight
- 2 bay leaves
- 3 cups chicken broth
- 1 can diced tomatoes

Instructions
1. Without the lid on, press the Sauté button on the Instant Pot.
2. Add the oil and sauté the chorizo for 2 minutes until crispy on the edges.
3. Stir in the onions and garlic until fragrant.
4. Add the rest of the ingredients.
5. Close the lid.
6. Press the Manual button and adjust the cooking time to 35 minutes.
7. Do natural pressure release.

Nutrition information:
Calories per serving: 392; Carbohydrates: 19.6g; Protein: 36.2g; Fat: 18.3g; Fiber: 6.1g

Simple Boiled Pinto Beans

Serves: 8
Preparation Time: 2 minutes
Cooking Time: 45 minutes
Ingredients
- 1-pound dry pinto beans, rinsed
- 5 ½ cups water
- 1 2/3 tablespoons vegetable bullion

Instructions
1. Place all ingredients in the Instant Pot.
2. Close the lid and seal off the vent.
3. Press the Manual button and adjust the cooking time to 45 minutes.

Nutrition information:
Calories per serving: 105; Carbohydrates: 14.8g; Protein: 5.1g; Fat: 3.2g; Fiber: 5.1g

Simple Boiled Kidney Beans

Serves: 2
Preparation Time: 2 minutes
Cooking Time: 40 minutes
Ingredients
- 1 cup dried white kidney beans
- ½ teaspoon salt
- 6 cups water

Instructions
1. Place all ingredients in the Instant Pot.
2. Close the lid and seal off the vent.
3. Press the Manual button and adjust the cooking time to 40 minutes.

Nutrition information:
Calories per serving: 56; Carbohydrates: 3.4g; Protein: 2.2g; Fat: 3.8g; Fiber: 0.1g

Black Eyed Peas and Ham

Serves: 10
Preparation Time: 2 minutes
Cooking Time: 30 minutes
Ingredients
- 1-pound dried black-eyed peas
- 6 ½ cups chicken stock
- 5 ounces ham, diced

Instructions
1. Place all ingredients in the Instant Pot.
2. Close the lid and seal off the vent.
3. Press the Manual button and adjust the cooking time to 30 minutes.

Nutrition information:
Calories per serving: 90; Carbohydrates: 9.1g; Protein: 7.6g; Fat: 2.4g; Fiber: 1.2g

Simple Spiced Black Beans

Serves: 12
Preparation Time: 2 minutes
Cooking Time: 30 minutes
Ingredients
- 2 ½ tablespoons vegetable bullion
- 1-pound dry black beans, rinsed
- 5 ½ cups water
- ½ teaspoon garlic powder
- ½ teaspoon coriander
- ½ teaspoon cumin
- ½ teaspoon paprika

Instructions
1. Place all ingredients in the Instant Pot.
2. Close the lid and seal off the vents.
3. Press the Manual button and adjust the cooking time to 30 minutes.

Nutrition information:
Calories per serving: 74; Carbohydrates: 9.4g; Protein: 3.1g; Fat: 3g; Fiber: 3.2g

Instant Pot Easy Baked Beans

Serves: 10
Preparation Time:
Cooking Time: 60 minutes
Ingredients
- 1-pound dry navy beans, soaked overnight
- 1 ½ tablespoons salt
- 6 cups water
- 6 strips of bacon, chopped
- 1 onion, chopped
- 2 cloves of garlic, chopped
- ¼ cup molasses
- 1 tablespoon soy sauce
- 3 bay leaves
- 2 teaspoons Dijon mustard
- 1 teaspoon apple cider vinegar
- Salt and pepper to taste

Instructions
1. Place the beans, 1 ½ tablespoons salt, and water in the Instant Pot.
2. Close the lid and press the Manual button. Adjust the cooking time to 30 minutes.

3. Once done, do natural release and drain the beans and set aside.
4. Without the lid on, press the Sauté button and add the bacon, onion, and garlic. Cook until the bacon has rendered, and the onion and garlic become aromatic.
5. Add the beans and the rest of the ingredients.
6. Close the lid and press the Manual button. Adjust the cooking time to 30 minutes.
7. Do natural pressure release.
Nutrition information:
Calories per serving: 56; Carbohydrates: 10.6g; Protein: 1.2g; Fat: 1.5g; Fiber: 1.3g

Greek Gigante Beans

Serves: 5
Preparation Time: 5 minutes
Cooking Time: 30 minutes
Ingredients
- 3 cups dried Gigantes beans
- 8 cups water
- 1 ½ teaspoon salt
- ¼ cup extra virgin olive oil
- 1 clove of garlic, minced
- 1 onion, chopped
- 1 stalk of celery, chopped
- 1 can crushed tomatoes
- 1 teaspoon dried oregano
- ½ cup water
- ½ cup feta cheese, crumbled

Instructions
1. Place the beans, water, and salt in the Instant Pot.
2. Close the lid and press the Manual button. Adjust the cooking time to 15 minutes.
3. Once done, drain the beans then set aside. Clean the inner pot and place it back into the Instant Pot.
4. Press the Sauté button and heat the oil. Stir in the garlic, onions, and celery. Stir until fragrant.
5. Add in the beans, crushed tomatoes, and oregano. Pour in the water.
6. Close the lid and press the Manual button. Cook for another 15 minutes.
7. Do natural pressure release.
8. Top with feta cheese.
Nutrition information:
Calories per serving: 115; Carbohydrates: 8.1g; Protein: 3.9g; Fat: 8.1g; Fiber: 3g

15-Bean Soup

Serves: 10
Preparation Time: 5 minutes
Cooking Time: 30 minutes
Ingredients
- 1 bag of 15-bean soup blend (Hurst Beans brand)
- 8 cups vegetable stock
- 3 cloves of garlic, minced
- 1 onion, chopped
- 1 red bell pepper, chopped
- 2 stalks of celery, chopped
- 2 carrots, peeled and chopped
- Salt and pepper to taste
- 1 bay leaf
- 3 sprigs of fresh thyme
- 1 can crushed tomatoes

- 1 tablespoon olive oil

Instructions
1. Place all ingredients in the Instant Pot.
2. Close the lid and seal off the vent.
3. Press the Manual button and adjust the cooking time to 30 minutes.
Nutrition information:
Calories per serving: 67; Carbohydrates: 11.6g; Protein: 2.5g; Fat: 2.1g; Fiber: 2.1g

Instant Pot Refried Beans

Serves: 2
Preparation Time: 5 minutes
Cooking Time: 60 minutes
Ingredients
- 1 cup pinto beans, drained and rinsed
- 3 cups water
- 3 tablespoons oil
- 2 cloves of garlic, chopped
- 1 onion, chopped
- 1 jalapeno pepper, chopped
- 1 bay leaf
- 1 tablespoon salt

Instructions
1. Place the beans and water in the Instant Pot. Close the lid and press the Manual button. Cook for 40 minutes.
2. Once done, do natural pressure release and drain the beans. Save the bean water.
3. Press the Sauté button on the Instant Pot and add the oil.
4. Stir in the garlic, onion, and jalapeno until fragrant.
5. Add the beans and the bean water.
6. Stir in the bay leaf and season with salt.
7. Close the lid and press the Manual button. Cook for another 20 minutes.
Nutrition information:
Calories per serving: 331; Carbohydrates: 29g; Protein: 8.6g; Fat: 21.1g; Fiber: 8.1g

13-Bean Soup

Serves: 4
Preparation Time: 2 minutes
Cooking Time: 30 minutes
Ingredients
- 1 ½ cups 13-bean soup mix
- 1 ham, diced
- 1 onion, chopped
- 1 tomatoes
- 2 teaspoons chili powder
- Salt and pepper to taste

Instructions
1. Place all ingredients in the Instant Pot.
2. Close the lid and seal off the vent.
3. Press the Manual button and adjust the cooking time to 30 minutes.
Nutrition information:
Calories per serving: 133; Carbohydrates: 13.4g; Protein: 14.5g; Fat: 2.9g; Fiber: 3.6g

Lazy Man's Baked Beans

Serves: 6
Preparation Time: 5 minutes

Cooking Time: 60 minutes
Ingredients
- 1-pound white beans, rinsed
- 1 onion, minced
- 2 cloves of garlic, chopped
- ½ cup molasses
- ½ cup maple syrup
- 1/8 cup balsamic vinegar
- 1 tablespoon mustard powder
- 4 cups water
- Salt and pepper to taste

Instructions
1. Place all ingredients in the Instant Pot.
2. Give a good stir and close the lid to seal off the vents
3. Press the Bean/Chili button.
4. Adjust the cooking time to 60 minutes.
5. Do natural pressure release.

Nutrition information:
Calories per serving:420; Carbohydrates:88g; Protein: 18.2g; Fat: 0.8g; Fiber: 12g

Easy Lazy Pressure Cooker Chili

Serves: 6
Preparation Time: 3 minutes
Cooking Time: 40 minutes
Ingredients
- 7 cups beef broth
- ½ pounds kidney beans, rinsed
- 1-pound ground beef
- 1 medium white onion, diced
- 1 green bell pepper, diced
- 3 cloves of garlic, chopped
- 1 can diced tomatoes
- 1/4 cup tomato paste
- Salt and pepper to taste

Instructions
1. Place all ingredients in the Instant Pot and give a good stir.
2. Close the lid and seal off the vent.
3. Press the Bean/Chili button and cook on pre-set cooking time.
4. Do natural pressure release.

Nutrition information:
Calories per serving: 337; Carbohydrates: 30.4g; Protein: 22.6g; Fat: 13.9g; Fiber: 1.6g

Pumpkin Lentil Soup

Serves: 6
Preparation Time: 2 minutes
Cooking Time:40 minutes
Ingredients
- 8 cups water
- ½ pound lentils, rinsed
- 1 whole cooking pumpkin (around 4 cups)
- 1 cup diced onions
- 2 cloves of garlic, minced
- 2 teaspoons allspice
- ¼ teaspoon cinnamon
- ¼ teaspoon cayenne
- ½ teaspoon nutmeg
- ½ cup heavy cream
- 1 tablespoon olive oil
- Salt and pepper to taste

Instructions
1. Place all ingredients in the Instant Pot.
2. Stir to combine everything.
3. Close the lid and make sure that the vent is sealed.
4. Press the Bean/Chili button and cook on pre-set cooking time.
5. Once cooked, place all ingredients in the blender and pulse until smooth.

Nutrition information:
Calories per serving: 123; Carbohydrates: 12.2g; Protein: 5.1g; Fat: 7.2g; Fiber: 1.2g

Instant Pot Green Split Pea Soup

Serves: 6
Preparation Time: 2 minutes
Cooking Time:40 minutes
Ingredients
- 1-pound green split peas
- 6 cups of beef broth
- 1 cup chopped carrots
- 1 cup chopped celery
- 1 cup onion
- 1 clove of garlic, minced
- 1 cup leftover ham, chopped
- Salt and pepper to taste

Instructions
1. Place all ingredients in the Instant Pot.
2. Give a good stir to mix everything.
3. Close the lid and make sure that the vent is sealed.
4. Press the Bean/Chili button.
5. Cook using the preset setting.
6. Do natural pressure release.

Nutrition information:
Calories per serving: 246; Carbohydrates: 41.5g; Protein: 11.5g; Fat: 4.2g; Fiber: 7.7g

15-Bean Tailgate Chili in Instant Pot

Serves: 6
Preparation Time: 2 minutes
Cooking Time: 40 minutes
Ingredients
- 1 can 15-bean soup
- ½ pound kidney beans, rinsed
- 1-pound ground sausage
- 1-pound ground sirloin
- 1-pound chuck roast, cubed
- 3 cups chopped onion
- 5 cloves of garlic, minced
- 2 poblano chilies, chopped
- 2 Anaheim chilies, chopped
- 5 cups beef stock
- 1 can diced tomatoes
- 1 can crushed tomatoes
- 2 tablespoons ground chipotle powder
- ½ tablespoon cumin
- ½ tablespoon allspice
- Salt and pepper to taste

Instructions
1. Place all ingredients in the Instant Pot.
2. Give a good stir to mix everything.
3. Close the lid and make sure that the vent is sealed.
4. Press the Bean/Chili button.

5. Cook using the preset setting.
6. Do natural pressure release.
Nutrition information:
Calories per serving: 503; Carbohydrates: 22.6g; Protein: 58.8g; Fat: 20.4g; Fiber: 6.1g

Instant Pot Hummus

Serves: 6 minutes
Preparation Time: 5 minutes
Cooking Time: 60 minutes
Ingredients
- 3 ½ cups water
- ½ teaspoon garlic powder
- ½ teaspoon salt
- ½ pounds dry garbanzo beans --
- 1/3 cup tahini
- Zest of ½ lemon
- Juice of 1 whole lemon
- 2 tablespoons olive oil
- ¾ teaspoon salt
- ¼ teaspoon pepper
- ¼ teaspoon cumin
- 1 clove of garlic minced
- A dash of paprika

Instructions
1. Place the water, garlic powder, salt, and garbanzo beans in the Instant Pot.
2. Close the lid and seal off the vent.
3. Press the Bean/Chili button and adjust the cooking time to 60 minutes.
4. Do natural pressure release.
5. Drain the beans and reserve 1/3 of the liquid.
6. Place the beans and the rest of the ingredients including the reserved 1/3 bean liquid in a food processor.
7. Pulse until smooth.
8. Place on a serving bowl.
9. Add a dash of olive oil and paprika on top.
Nutrition information:
Calories per serving:265; Carbohydrates: 27.4g; Protein: 10.1g; Fat: 13.9g; Fiber: 5.9g

Instant Pot Red Beans and Rice

Serves: 10
Preparation Time: 5 minutes
Cooking Time: 50 minutes
Ingredients
- 1 medium onion, diced
- 1 bell pepper, diced
- 3 stalks of celery, diced
- 3 cloves of garlic, minced
- 1-pound red kidney beans
- Salt and pepper to taste
- 1 teaspoon fresh thyme
- 2 bay leaves
- 7 cups water
- 1-pound andouille sausage, sliced
- 10 cups cooked rice

Instructions
1. Place all ingredients in the Instant Pot except for the cooked rice.
2. Close the lid and seal off the vent.
3. Press the Bean/Chili button.
4. Cook for 50 minutes until the beans are soft.
5. Do natural pressure release.
6. Once cooked, mix in the rice until well-combined.
Nutrition information:
Calories per serving: 536; Carbohydrates: 72.2g; Protein: 26.9g; Fat:33.1 g; Fiber: 28.9g

Instant Pot Ham and Bean Soup

Serves: 6
Preparation Time: 5 minutes
Cooking Time: 50 minutes
Ingredients
- 1-pound white beans, rinsed
- 8 cups chicken broth
- 1 leftover ham bone with meat
- 1 onion diced
- 1 clove of garlic, minced
- 1 teaspoon chili powder
- 1 can diced tomatoes
- 1 lemon, juiced

Instructions
1. Place all ingredients in the Instant Pot.
2. Give a good stir to mix everything.
3. Close the lid and make sure that the vent is sealed.
4. Press the Bean/Chili button.
5. Adjust the cooking time to 50 minutes.
6. Do natural pressure release.
Nutrition information:
Calories per serving: 788; Carbohydrates: 54.3g; Protein: 88.3g; Fat: 23.1g; Fiber: 12.8g

Instant Pot Drunken Beans

Serves: 8
Preparation Time: 3 minutes
Cooking Time: 1 hour
Ingredients
- 6 slices of bacon, cut into ¼-inch pieces
- 1 cup onion, diced
- 1 cup green pepper, diced
- 3 cloves of garlic, minced
- 1-pound Pinto beans, rinsed
- 1 can crushed tomatoes
- 12 ounces Mexican beer or any beer of your choice
- 2 cups chicken stock
- 1 teaspoon cumin
- Salt and pepper to taste

Instructions
1. Without the lid on, press the Sauté button on the Instant Pot and add the bacon and onions. Sauté for a minute until the onions are fragrant.
2. Add the green pepper and garlic and sauté for 30 seconds.
3. Pour in the rest of the ingredients.
4. Close the lid and seal off the vent.
5. Press the Bean/Chili button and adjust the cooking time to 50 minutes.
6. Once the timer beeps, do natural pressure release.
Nutrition information:
Calories per serving: 464; Carbohydrates: 42.1g; Protein: 26.8g; Fat: 21.4g; Fiber: 9.7g

Tex-Mex Pinto Beans

Serves: 4

Preparation Time: 5 minutes
Cooking Time: 50 minutes
Ingredients
- ½ pound pinto beans
- 5 cups chicken broth
- 1 onion, chopped
- 1 jalapeno, chopped
- 1 clove of garlic, minced
- 1 pack taco seasoning
- ½ cup Salsa Verde
- Salt and pepper to taste
- ¼ cup cilantro, chopped

Instructions
1. Place all ingredients in the Instant Pot except for cilantro.
2. Give a good stir to mix everything.
3. Close the lid and make sure that the vent is sealed.
4. Press the Bean/Chili button.
5. Adjust the cooking time to 50 minutes.
6. Do natural pressure release.
7. Garnish with cilantro and serve on top of rice or taco shells.

Nutrition information:
Calories per serving: 699; Carbohydrates: 43.6g; Protein: 77.9g; Fat: 21.8g; Fiber: 10g

Beans with Cajun Sausages Soup

Serves: 8
Preparation Time: 2 minutes
Cooking Time: 50 minutes
Ingredients
- ½ pound white beans, rinsed
- 1 green bell pepper, diced
- 1 onion, diced
- 8 cups chicken broth
- ½ pound andouille sausages
- 1 can diced tomatoes
- ½ teaspoon garlic powder
- ½ teaspoon paprika
- ½ teaspoon onion powder
- ½ teaspoon cayenne pepper
- ½ teaspoon dried thyme
- ½ teaspoon oregano
- Salt and pepper to taste

Instructions
1. Place all ingredients in the Instant Pot.
2. Give a good stir to mix everything.
3. Close the lid and make sure that the vent is sealed.
4. Press the Bean/Chili button.
5. Adjust the cooking time to 50 minutes.
6. Do natural pressure release.

Nutrition information:
Calories per serving:562; Carbohydrates: 25.3g; Protein: 64.4g; Fat: 22.3g; Fiber: 6.1g

Sweet and Savory Baked Beans

Serves: 10
Preparation Time: 5 minutes
Cooking Time: 50 minutes
Ingredients
- 1-pound navy beans
- 1 onion, chopped
- 2 cloves of garlic, minced
- 2 cups hot water
- 1/3 cup dates, chopped
- ¼ cup maple syrup
- 1 tablespoon soy sauce
- 1 teaspoon dry mustard
- 1 teaspoon ginger, grated
- ¼ teaspoon red pepper
- 20 ounces crushed pineapples, juice included
- ¼ cup tomato paste
- 1 tablespoon molasses
- 1 tablespoon cider vinegar
- 1 teaspoon onion powder
- ½ teaspoon garlic powder
- ¼ teaspoon liquid smoke
- Salt and pepper to taste

Instructions
1. Place all ingredients in the Instant Pot.
2. Give a good stir to mix everything.
3. Close the lid and make sure that the vent is sealed.
4. Press the Bean/Chili button.
5. Adjust the cooking time to 50 minutes.
6. Do natural pressure release.

Nutrition information:
Calories per serving: 243; Carbohydrates: 50g; Protein: 11g; Fat: 0.7g; Fiber: 9g

Instant Pot Cuban Black Beans

Serves: 6
Preparation Time: 5 minutes
Cooking Time:50 minutes
Ingredients
- ½ pounds black beans, rinsed
- 1 teaspoon olive oil
- 2 cup smoked ham hock, chopped
- ½ cup onion, chopped
- 2 green pepper, seeded then chopped
- 4 cloves of garlic, minced
- 2 tablespoons tomato paste
- 2 ½ teaspoons ground cumin
- 1 teaspoon sugar
- 6 cups water
- Salt and pepper to taste

Instructions
1. Place all ingredients in the Instant Pot.
2. Give a good stir to mix everything.
3. Close the lid and make sure that the vent is sealed.
4. Press the Bean/Chili button.
5. Adjust the cooking time to 50 minutes.
6. Do natural pressure release.
7. Serve over rice.

Nutrition information:
Calories per serving: 246; Carbohydrates: 29.8g; Protein: 23.3g; Fat: 4.4g; Fiber: 6.7g

Indian Green Beans and Potatoes

Serves: 3
Preparation Time: 8 minutes
Cooking Time: 25 minutes
Ingredients
- 1 tablespoon oil
- ½ teaspoon cumin seed
- 2 teaspoon coriander powder
- ¼ teaspoon turmeric

- 4 cloves of garlic, chopped
- 1 green chili, chopped
- 2 cups green beans
- 1 potato, cubed
- ¼ teaspoon salt
- 1 teaspoon dry mango powder or amchur powder
- Salt to taste

Instructions
1. Without the lid on, press the Sauté button on the Instant Pot.
2. Add in the oil and wait until it heats up. Add the cumin seeds and fry for 1 minute or until they pop.
3. Stir in the coriander, turmeric, and garlic. Stir until the garlic is fragrant.
4. Pour in the rest of the ingredients.
5. Stir to combine.
6. Close the lid and seal off the vent.
7. Press the Manual button and adjust the cooking time to 25 minutes.
8. Do natural pressure release.

Nutrition information:
Calories per serving:166; Carbohydrates: 27.8g; Protein: 3.9g; Fat: 5.2g; Fiber: 4.8g

Brothy Beans with Cream

Serves: 4
Preparation Time: 5 minutes
Cooking Time: 50 minutes

Ingredients
- 2 cups mixed dried heirloom beans, soaked overnight
- 2 quarts chicken stock
- 4 sprigs thyme
- Salt and pepper to taste
- ½ cup heavy cream

Instructions
1. Place all ingredients in the Instant Pot except for the cream.
2. Close the lid and press the Manual button.
3. Adjust the cooking time to 45 minutes.
4. Do quick pressure release.
5. Without the lid on, press the Sauté button and add in the heavy cream.
6. Allow to simmer for 5 minutes.

Nutrition information:
Calories per serving:619; Carbohydrates: 8.1g; Protein: 98.8g; Fat: 18.6g; Fiber: 3g

Navy Bean Escarole Stew

Serves: 6
Preparation Time: 5 minutes
Cooking Time: 50 minutes

Ingredients
- 6 tablespoons olive oil
- 1 bulb of garlic, minced and divided
- 1 onion, chopped
- 1 small fennel, chopped
- 1 tablespoon grated lemon zest
- 2 teaspoons rosemary, chopped
- ½ teaspoon red pepper flakes
- 2 bay leaves
- 2 cups dried navy beans, rinsed
- 6 cups chicken broth
- salt to taste
- 8 ounces feta cheese
- 4 large sprigs of basil
- 1 cup olives, pitted
- 1 head of escarole
- 3 tablespoon fresh lemon juice

Instructions
1. Press the Sauté button on the Instant Pot.
2. Sauté the garlic, onion, and fennel until fragrant.
3. Add the lemon zest, rosemary, red pepper flakes, bay leaves, navy beans, chicken broth, and salt.
4. Close the lid and secure the vent.
5. Press the Manual button and adjust the cooking time to 50 minutes.
6. Once the timer beeps, do quick pressure release.
7. Without the lid on, press the Sauté button and add in the feta cheese, basil, olive, escarole and lemon juice.
8. Simmer for 3 minutes before serving.

Nutrition information:
Calories per serving:869; Carbohydrates: 49.7g; Protein: 73.2g; Fat: 41.6g; Fiber: 11.8g

Sausage Greens and Bean Pasta

Serves: 5
Preparation Time: 4 minutes
Cooking Time: 20 minutes

Ingredients
- 2 tablespoons olive oil
- 2 sprigs of rosemary
- 1 cup Italian sausage, ground
- 1 can chickpeas, rinsed
- ¼ cup dry white wine
- 12 ounces pasta of your choice
- ½ cup chicken broth
- Salt and pepper to taste
- ½ cup parmesan cheese, grated
- 2 tablespoons butter

Instructions
1. Press the Sauté button on the Instant Pot and add the olive oil.
2. Stir in the rosemary and sausages. Cook until the sausages turn slightly brown.
3. Add the chickpeas, white wine, pasta, and chicken broth. Season with salt and pepper to taste.
4. Close the lid and press the Manual button.
5. Adjust the cooking time to 20 minutes.
6. Do quick pressure release.
7. Garnish with parmesan cheese and allow butter to melt on top.
8. Serve.

Nutrition information:
Calories per serving: 407; Carbohydrates: 33g; Protein: 17.4g; Fat: 23.5g; Fiber:6.6 g

Cannellini Beans with Shrimp and Tomatoes

Serves: 6
Preparation Time: 2 minutes
Cooking Time: 18 minutes

Ingredients
- 4 tablespoons olive oil
- 1 shallots chopped

- 2 chilies, chopped
- 4 cloves of garlic, minced
- 1 can cannellini beans, rinsed
- 1 can cherry tomatoes
- 1 tablespoon red wine vinegar
- 3 cups chicken broth
- Salt and pepper to taste
- 1-pound shrimps, peeled and deveined
- ½ cup olives pitted
- Basil leaves for garnish

Instructions
1. Press the Sauté button on the Instant Pot and heat the oil.
2. Sauté the shallots, chilies, and garlic until fragrant.
3. Add the beans, cherry tomatoes, red wine vinegar, and broth. Season with salt and pepper to taste.
4. Close the lid and seal off the vent.
5. Press the Manual button and adjust the cooking time to 15 minutes.
6. Do natural pressure release.
7. Open the lid and add the shrimps and olives.
8. Press the Sauté button and allow to simmer for 3 minutes to cook the shrimps.
9. Garnish with basil leaves.

Nutrition information:
Calories per serving: 366; Carbohydrates: 3.5g; Protein: 41.8g; Fat: g19.5; Fiber: 0.6g

Spice Bean and Chicken Chorizo Chili

Serves: 5
Preparation Time: 6 minutes
Cooking Time: 15 minutes

Ingredients
- 3 tablespoons olive oil
- 1 ½ pounds chicken chorizo, sliced
- 1 onion, chopped
- 2 cloves of garlic
- 1 cup beer or lager
- 1/3 cup chili powder
- 1 can black beans, rinsed
- 1 tablespoon oregano
- ¼ teaspoon ground cinnamon
- 2 bay leaves
- 1 can diced tomatoes
- 2 cups chicken broth
- Salt and pepper to taste

Instructions
1. Press the Sauté button on the Instant Pot.
2. Heat the oil and stir in the chicken chorizo, onion, and garlic until fragrant and slightly brown.
3. Stir in the rest of the ingredients.
4. Close the lid and seal off the vent.
5. Press the Manual button and adjust the cooking time to 15 minutes.
6. Do natural pressure release.

Nutrition information:
Calories per serving:704; Carbohydrates:59.8 g; Protein: 67.3g; Fat: 20.8g; Fiber: 16.3g

Mixed Beans Salad

Serves: 6
Preparation Time: 3 minutes
Cooking Time: 50 minutes

Ingredients
- 1 cup black beans, dry
- 1 cup kidney beans, dry
- 1 cup red beans, dry
- 6 cups chicken stock
- Salt and pepper to taste
- 1 teaspoon oregano
- 5 plum tomatoes, chopped
- ½ red onion chopped
- 2 serrano chilies, chopped
- ½ cup cilantro leaves, chopped
- ¼ cup olive oil

Instructions
1. Place the beans, chicken stock, salt, and pepper in the Instant Pot.
2. Close the lid and seal off the vent.
3. Press the Manual button and adjust the cooking time to 50 minutes.
4. Do natural pressure release.
5. Drain the beans from the liquid and allow to cool completely.
6. Assemble the salad by combining the rest of the ingredients in a bowl including the beans.
7. Season with salt and pepper to taste.

Nutrition information:
Calories per serving: 436; Carbohydrates: 58.3g; Protein: 20.9g; Fat: 14.1g; Fiber: 10.3g

Black Bean Soup with Poblano Chilies

Serves: 6
Preparation Time: 3 minutes
Cooking Time:50 minutes

Ingredients
- 2 poblano chilies, chopped
- 2 tablespoons pepitas or pumpkin seeds, shelled
- 1 large ancho chili, chopped
- 1 tablespoon vegetable oil
- 1 onion, chopped
- 4 cloves of garlic, minced
- 1 can diced tomatoes
- 4 cups chicken broth
- 2 cans black beans, drained and rinsed
- Salt and pepper to taste
- ½ cup feta cheese, crumbled
- Lime wedges for garnish

Instructions
1. Place all ingredients in the Instant Pot except for the cream.
2. Close the lid and press the Manual button.
3. Adjust the cooking time to 50 minutes.
4. Do quick pressure release.

Nutrition information:
Calories per serving: 453; Carbohydrates: 27.3g; Protein: 45.8g; Fat: 17.8g; Fiber: 8.7g

Butter Bean Ragout

Serves: 6
Preparation Time: 20 minutes
Cooking Time: 60 minutes

Ingredients
- 1 ¼ cups olive oil
- 2 cloves of garlic, minced
- 1 onion, chopped

- ½ small fennel bulb, chopped
- ¼ large celery root, peeled and cut into strips
- 1-pound dried butter bean, soaked overnight and drained
- ¾ parsley, chopped
- 2 bay leaves
- 1 cup chicken broth
- Salt to taste
- 3 cups Tuscan kale, chopped
- ½ cup panko breadcrumbs

Instructions
1. Without the lid on, press the Sauté button on the Instant Pot and pour the oil.
2. Once the oil is hot, sauté the garlic and onions until fragrant.
3. Stir in the fennel and celery root and sauté for another minute before adding the butter beans.
4. Stir in the parsley, bay leaves, and chicken broth. Season with salt and pepper.
5. Close the lid and press the Manual button and adjust the cooking time for 50 minutes.
6. Do quick natural release to open the lid.
7. Add the kale and panko breadcrumbs. Give a stir. Press the Sauté button and continue simmering for 3 minutes.
8. Serve warm.

Nutrition information:
Calories per serving:505; Carbohydrates: 19.9g; Protein: 6.4g; Fat: 45.8g; Fiber: 5.6g

Spicy Beans with Wilted Greens

Serves: 7
Preparation Time:
Cooking Time:

Ingredients
- ¼ cup olive oil
- 4 cloves of garlic, minced
- 1 onion, chopped
- 4 anchovy fillets
- 4 chilies, chopped
- 4 stalks of celery, chopped
- 1 sprig of rosemary
- 1-pound dried white beans, soaked overnight
- 1 cup chicken broth
- Salt and pepper to taste
- 1 bunch kale or mustard greens, chopped
- 1 bunch spinach, chopped
- 4 cups arugula, trimmed and chopped
- 2 teaspoons fresh lemon juice
- ½ cup parmesan, grated

Instructions
1. Press the Sauté button on the Instant Pot and pour the oil.
2. Sauté the garlic and onion until fragrant.
3. Add in the anchovy fillets, chilies, celery, and rosemary. Continue stirring until fragrant.
4. Stir in the beans and add the broth. Season with salt and pepper to taste.
5. Close the lid and make sure that the vent is set to sealing.
6. Press the Manual button and adjust the cooking time to 50 minutes.
7. Do natural pressure release.
8. Once the lid is open, press the Sauté button and add the green vegetables. Continue stirring for 2 minutes or until the veggies have wilted.
9. Add the lemon juice and grated parmesan.

Nutrition information:
Calories per serving:304; Carbohydrates: 42.3g; Protein: 18.2g; Fat: 8.1g; Fiber: 11.1g

Cannellini Beans Stew with Chicken and Dried Cherries

Serves: 6
Preparation Time: 5 minutes
Cooking Time: 20 minutes

Ingredients
- 6 tablespoons olive oil
- 1 cup shredded chicken meat
- 1 onion, chopped
- 2 teaspoons chili powder
- 1 teaspoon sambal oelek
- 2 tablespoons fish sauce
- 2 cans cannellini beans, drained and rinsed
- ½ cup dried cherries
- 2 cups chicken broth
- Salt and pepper to taste
- 2 tablespoons chopped parsley

Instructions
1. Without the lid on, press the Sauté button.
2. Pour the olive oil and sauté the chicken meat, onions, chili powder, and sambal oelek. Season with fish sauce.
3. Stir in the cannellini beans and cherries.
4. Add the broth and season with salt and pepper.
5. Close the lid and seal the vent.
6. Press the Manual button and adjust the cooking time to 20 minutes.
7. Do natural pressure release and garnish with parsley.

Nutrition information:
Calories per serving: 340; Carbohydrates: 24.3g; Protein: 17.1g; Fat: 19.7g; Fiber: 6.3g

Cannellini and Tomato Soup

Serves: 8
Preparation Time: 5 minutes
Cooking Time: 50 minutes

Ingredients
- 4 tablespoons olive oil
- 1 onion, quartered
- 4 cloves of garlic, crushed
- 1 fennel bulb, chopped
- 1 tablespoon Sherry vinegar
- 1 cup dried cannellini beans, soaked overnight
- 2 bay leaves
- 1 can tomatoes, peeled
- ½ teaspoon red pepper flakes
- 4 cups vegetable broth
- Salt to taste
- 1 bunch Swiss chard, chopped

Instructions
1. Without the lid on, press the Sauté button on the Instant Pot.
2. Pour in the oil and sauté the onion, garlic and fennel bulbs until fragrant.

3. Stir in the sherry vinegar, beans, bay leaves, tomatoes, red pepper flakes, and broth.
4. Season with salt and pepper to taste.
5. Close the lid and press the Manual button.
6. Adjust the cooking time to 50 minutes.
7. Do natural pressure release.
8. Once the lid is open, press the Sauté button and add the greens.
9. Simmer until the vegetables have wilted.

Nutrition information:
Calories per serving:92; Carbohydrates: 7.4g; Protein: 1.1g; Fat: 6.9g; Fiber: 2g

Spicy Bean Soup with Sausages

Serves: 8
Preparation Time: 4 minutes
Cooking Time: 25 minutes

Ingredients
- 2 tablespoons olive oil
- 1-pound sausages, chopped
- 1 onion, chopped
- 4 cloves of garlic, minced
- 1 tablespoon rosemary, chopped
- ¼ teaspoon red pepper flakes
- 4 cups chicken stock
- 3 cans cannellini beans, drained and rinsed
- 2 large sweet peppers, chopped
- 3 carrots, chopped
- Salt and pepper to taste
- ½ cup almond milk
- 1-pound baby spinach, shredded
- ¼ cup parmesan cheese, grated

Instructions
1. Without the lid on, press the Sauté button on the Instant Pot and pour in the olive oil.
2. Add the sausages, onion, and garlic. Cook for 3 minutes or until fragrant
3. Add the rosemary, red pepper flakes, and chicken stock. Scrape the bottom to remove the browning.
4. Stir in the beans, sweet peppers, and carrots. Season with salt and pepper to taste.
5. Close the lid and seal off the vent.
6. Press the Manual button and adjust the cooking time to 20 minutes.
7. Do quick natural release.
8. Once the lid is open, press the Sauté button again and add in the almond milk and baby spinach. Stir and allow to simmer for 5 minutes.
9. Sprinkle with parmesan cheese on top.

Nutrition information:
Calories per serving: 409; Carbohydrates: 41.2g; Protein:23.7g; Fat:18.9g; Fiber: 10.1g

Pasta Cannellini with Escarole

Serves: 5
Preparation Time: 5 minutes
Cooking Time: 20 minutes

Ingredients
- 1 ½ cups canned cannellini beans, rinsed
- 2 carrots, chopped into large pieces
- 2 celery stalks, chopped
- 1 bulb of garlic, minced
- 6 sprigs of parsley
- 1 sprig of rosemary
- 2 bay leaves
- 1 onion, chopped
- 1 can crushed tomatoes
- ¾ cup dry white wine
- 3 ounces pasta of your choice
- Salt and pepper to taste
- ½ small head of escarole, torn
- 3 tablespoons olive oil

Instructions
1. Place all ingredients except for the olive oil and escarole in the Instant Pot.
2. Give a stir to mix everything.
3. Close the lid and secure the vent.
4. Press the Manual button and adjust the cooking time to 15 minutes.
5. Do manual pressure release for 5 minutes.
6. Open the lid and press the Sauté button.
7. Stir in the escarole leaves and cook for 2 minutes until wilted.
8. Drizzle with olive oil last.

Nutrition information:
Calories per serving: 231; Carbohydrates: 22.8g; Protein: 8.66g; Fat: 12.9g; Fiber: 3g

Mexican Beans with Beef Soup

Serves: 7
Preparation Time: 5 minutes
Cooking Time: 50 minutes

Ingredients
- 2 tablespoons vegetable oil
- 4 slices bacon
- 1 ½ pounds flank steak
- 2 cloves of garlic, minced
- 4 tomatillos, husks removed then rinsed
- 4 serrano chilies, seeds removed and chopped
- 6 cups beef stock
- 3 cups dried pinto beans, soaked overnight
- Salt and pepper to taste
- ½ cup cilantro, chopped
- 6 spring onions, chopped

Instructions
1. Press the Sauté button on the Instant Pot and add the oil.
2. Add the bacon, flank steak, and garlic. Sauté for a few minutes until the bacon renders oil and the garlic turns brown.
3. Stir in the tomatillos and Serrano. Stir for a few minutes.
4. Pour in the beef stock and the dried pinto beans. Season with salt and pepper to taste.
5. Close the lid and seal off the vent.
6. Press the Manual button and adjust the cooking time to 50 minutes.
7. Do a quick pressure release.
8. While still hot, add the cilantro and spring onions.

Nutrition information:
Calories per serving: 555; Carbohydrates: 57.4g; Protein: 45.1g; Fat: 16.2g; Fiber: 13.7g

Gigante Beans in Tomato Sauce

Serves: 8
Preparation Time: 3 minutes

Cooking Time: 50 minutes
Ingredients
- ¼ cup olive oil
- 1 onion, chopped
- 4 cloves of garlic, sliced
- ½ teaspoon red pepper flakes, crushed
- ½ cup dry white wine
- 2 ½ cups dried Gigante beans, soaked overnight
- 2 bay leaves
- 1 can whole peeled tomatoes
- Salt and pepper to taste
- ½ cup feta cheese, crumbled

Instructions
1. Place all ingredients in the Instant Pot except for the feta cheese.
2. Close the lid and seal off the vent.
3. Press the Bean/Chili button and adjust the cooking time to 50 minutes.
4. Do natural pressure release.
5. Sprinkle with feta cheese before serving.

Nutrition information:
Calories per serving: 126; Carbohydrates: 5.1g; Protein: 3.8; Fat:10.5g; Fiber:1.3g

Baked with Beans with Bacon

Serves: 7
Preparation Time: 3 minutes
Cooking Time: 60 minutes
Ingredients
- 2 cups dried navy beans, soaked overnight then rinsed
- 2 onions, chopped
- 1 bulb garlic, minced
- 2 bay leaves
- 8 ounces slab of bacon, cut into pieces
- ¼ cup dry white wine
- 3 cups beef broth
- Salt and pepper to taste
- 2 tablespoons olive oil
- ½ cup parmesan cheese, grated

Instructions
1. Place all ingredients in the Instant Pot except for the olive oil and parmesan cheese.
2. Stir to combine everything.
3. Close the lid and seal off the vent.
4. Press the Bean/Chili button and adjust the cooking time to 1 hour.
5. Do natural pressure release.
6. Once the lid is open, drizzle with olive oil and sprinkle with parmesan cheese on top.

Nutrition information:
Calories per serving: 430; Carbohydrates: 51.6g; Protein:20.7 g; Fat: 17.3g; Fiber: 10.7g

Spicy Fava Bean Soup

Serves: 5
Preparation Time: 5 minutes
Cooking Time: 60 minutes
Ingredients
- ½ cup olive oil
- 2 onions, quartered
- 4 cloves of garlic, minced
- 1 can crushed tomatoes
- 2 teaspoons ground cumin
- ½ teaspoon ground coriander
- ¼ teaspoon ground allspice
- 8 cups vegetable broth
- 1 ½ cups dried fava beans, soaked overnight
- Salt and pepper to taste
- 1/3 cup plain Greek yogurt

Instructions
1. Without the lid on, press the Sauté button.
2. Pour in the oil and sauté the onions and garlic until fragrant.
3. Add the tomatoes, cumin, coriander, and allspice. Continue stirring for 3 minutes.
4. Pour in the broth and fava beans. Season with salt and pepper to taste.
5. Close the lid and seal off the vent.
6. Press the Manual button and adjust the cooking time to 50 minutes.
7. Do natural pressure release.
8. Once opened, stir in the Greek yogurt and press the Sauté button and allow to simmer for 3 minutes.

Nutrition information:
Calories per serving:284; Carbohydrates: 19.3g; Protein: 5.4g; Fat: 22.3g; Fiber: 4.6g

Beans and Squash Minestrone

Serves: 8
Preparation Time:5 minutes
Cooking Time:25 minutes
Ingredients
- ¼ cups olive oil
- 1 ½ pounds ham hocks, chopped
- 1 onion, chopped
- 2 cloves of garlic, minced
- 2 leeks white part only, chopped
- 2 stalks of celery, chopped
- 1 butternut squash, seeded and sliced into ½-inch pieces
- 1-pound green beans, cut into 1-inch pieces
- 2 cans navy beans, rinsed
- 1 cup small pasta shells
- 8 cups chicken broth
- Salt and pepper to taste
- 2 bunches flat-leaf spinach, chopped

Instructions
1. Press the Sauté button on the Instant Pot and pour the olive oil.
2. Sauté the ham hocks and add the onions and garlic. Stir until fragrant.
3. Add the leeks, celery, butternut squash, green beans, and navy beans. Stir for 30 seconds before pouring in the chicken broth.
4. Season with salt and pepper to taste.
5. Close the lid and seal off the vent.
6. Press the Manual button and adjust the cooking time to 20 minutes.
7. Do quick pressure release and add the spinach last.
8. Allow the spinach to cook in the soup's own heat.

Nutrition information:
Calories per serving:753; Carbohydrates: 49.1g; Protein: 80.6g; Fat: 27.1g; Fiber: 11.3g

White Beans and Broccoli

Serves: 7
Preparation Time: 5 minutes
Cooking Time: 25 minutes
Ingredients
- 3 tablespoons olive oil
- 2 anchovy fillets, packed in oil
- 4 cloves of garlic, sliced
- 2 cans cannellini beans, rinsed
- ¼ cup parsley, chopped
- 1 cup chicken broth
- Salt and pepper to taste
- 1 head broccoli, cut into florets
- 2 tablespoons parmesan cheese, grated

Instructions
1. Press the Sauté button on the Instant Pot.
2. Add the oil and sauté the anchovy fillets and garlic until fragrant.
3. Add the beans and parsley. Pour in the broth. Season with salt and pepper to taste
4. Close the lid and seal off the vent.
5. Press the Manual button and adjust the cooking time to 20 minutes.
6. Do natural pressure release.
7. Once the lid is open, press the Sauté button and add the broccoli florets. Stir and allow to simmer for 5 minutes until the vegetables are done.
8. Sprinkle with parmesan cheese.

Nutrition information:
Calories per serving: 66; Carbohydrates: 1.6g; Protein: 1.1g; Fat: 6.4g; Fiber: 1.3g

Italian Bean Stew

Serves: 9
Preparation Time: 5 minutes
Cooking Time: 25 minutes
Ingredients
- ½ cup olive oil
- 4 cloves of garlic, chopped
- ½ teaspoon red pepper flakes
- 2 medium carrots, chopped
- 2 stalks of celery, chopped
- 1 leek white part, chopped
- 1 can tomatoes
- 3 cans cannellini beans, rinsed
- 1 bay leaf
- 1 sprig thyme
- 5 cups chicken broth
- Salt and pepper to taste
- 1 bunch collard greens, chopped
- ½ cup parmesan cheese, grated

Instructions
1. Press the Sauté button and pour the olive oil.
2. Sauté the garlic, red pepper flakes, carrots, celery, and leeks until fragrant.
3. Add the tomatoes and beans.
4. Stir in the bay leaf, thyme, and chicken broth.
5. Season with salt and pepper to taste.
6. Close the lid and press the Manual button. Adjust the cooking time to 25 minutes.
7. Once cooked, do quick pressure release.
8. Open the lid and press the Sauté button.
9. Stir in the collard greens and allow to simmer for 3 minutes.
10. Sprinkle with parmesan cheese on top.

Nutrition information:
Calories per serving: 361; Carbohydrates: 6.6g; Protein:31.2 g; Fat: 22.9g; Fiber: 1.2g

Stewed Spicy Cannellini Beans

Serves: 8
Preparation Time: 5 minutes
Cooking Time: 50 minutes
Ingredients
- 1-pound dried cannellini beans, soaked overnight and rinsed
- 1 onion, halved
- 1 bulb garlic, minced
- 1 fennel bulb, sliced
- 1 carrot, peeled then chopped
- 4 sprigs of thyme
- 2 dried chilies
- 1/3 cup olive oil
- 6 cups chicken broth
- Salt and pepper to taste

Instructions
1. Place all ingredients in the Instant Pot.
2. Close the lid and seal off the vent.
3. Press the Bean/Chili button and adjust the cooking time to 50 minutes.
4. Do natural pressure release.

Nutrition information:
Calories per serving:111; Carbohydrates: 7.1g; Protein: 1.3g; Fat: 9.2g; Fiber: 2.5g

Grains Recipes

Instant Pot Rice

Serves: 8
Preparation Time: 5 minutes
Cooking Time: 25 minutes
Ingredients
- 3 cups rice (any type)
- 3 cups water
- A dash of salt

Instructions
1. Rinse the rice under cold running water.
2. Place the rice in the Instant Pot and pour in water.
3. Season with salt.
4. Close the lid and seal off the valve.
5. Press the Rice button and adjust the cooking time depending on the type of rice you are cooking.
6. If you are cooking for white rice, set the timer for 6 minutes and 22 minutes for brown rice.
7. Do natural pressure release.
8. Fluff the rice once cooked.

Nutrition information:
Calories per serving: 140; Carbohydrates: 21.9g; Protein: 5.9g; Fat: 9.3g; Fiber: 9.3g

Chicken and Rice

Serves: 6
Preparation Time: 5 minutes
Cooking Time: 15 minutes
Ingredients
- 1 tablespoon oil
- 3 small shallots, diced
- 2 cloves of garlic, minced
- 1-pound boneless chicken thighs
- Salt and pepper to taste
- 3 carrots, diced
- 1 ½ cups white jasmine rice, rinsed and drained
- 1 ½ cups chicken stock
- 2 tablespoons thyme leaves

Instructions
1. Press the Sauté button on the Instant Pot and pour in the oil
2. Sauté the shallots and garlic until fragrant.
3. Add in the chicken thighs and season with salt and pepper to taste. Continue stirring for 5 minutes until the chicken meat has browned a little.
4. Stir in the rest of the ingredients.
5. Close the lid and seal off the vent.
6. Press the Manual button and adjust the cooking time to 15 minutes.
7. Do natural pressure release

Nutrition information:
Calories per serving: 362; Carbohydrates: 47.3g; Protein: 21.5g; Fat: 9g; Fiber: 2.5g

Indian Vegetable Rice

Serves: 6
Preparation Time: 3 minutes
Cooking Time: 22 minutes
Ingredients
- 1 tablespoon olive oil
- ¼ cup shallots, chopped
- 1 clove of garlic, minced
- 1 ½ cups basmati rice, rinsed
- ½ cup carrots, chopped
- 2 teaspoons curry powder
- 2 cups chicken broth
- Salt and pepper to taste
- 1 cup frozen peas

Instructions
1. Heat the oil in the Instant Pot by pressing the Sauté button.
2. Sauté the shallots and garlic until fragrant.
3. Add the rest of the ingredients.
4. Give a stir and scrape the bottom of the pot.
5. Close the lid and seal off the vent.
6. Press the Rice button and adjust the cooking time to 20 minutes.
7. Do natural pressure release.

Nutrition information:
Calories per serving: 261; Carbohydrates: 19.5g; Protein: 22.3g; Fat: 14.4g; Fiber: 7.8g

Cilantro Lime Rice

Serves: 10
Preparation Time: 5 minutes
Cooking Time: 17 minutes
Ingredients
- 1 can vegetable broth
- ¾ cup water
- 2 tablespoons canola oil
- 3 tablespoons juice of lime juice
- 2 cups long grain white rice, rinsed
- Zest of 1 lime
- ½ cup cilantro, chopped
- ½ teaspoon salt

Instructions
1. Place everything in the pot and give a good stir.
2. Give a good stir and close the lid.
3. Seal off the vent.
4. Press the Rice button and adjust the cooking time to 17 minutes.
5. Do natural pressure release.
6. Fluff the rice before serving.

Nutrition information:
Calories per serving: 166; Carbohydrates: 31.2g; Protein: 2.7 g; Fat: 3.1g; Fiber: 0.5g

Instant Pot Spanish Rice

Serves: 8
Preparation Time: 5 minutes
Cooking Time: 20 minutes
Ingredients
- ½ onion, chopped
- ½ red bell pepper, chopped
- 1 ½ cups white rice, rinsed
- 2 cups vegetable broth
- ½ teaspoon chili powder
- ¼ teaspoon ground cumin
- 1 cup salsa

Instructions
1. Place everything in the pot and give a good stir.
2. Give a good stir and close the lid.
3. Seal off the vent.

4. Press the Rice button and adjust the cooking time to 20 minutes.
5. Do natural pressure release.
6. Fluff the rice before serving.
Nutrition information:
Calories per serving:145; Carbohydrates: 32.3g; Protein:3.3 g; Fat:0.3 g; Fiber: 1.8g

Instant Pot Rice Pilaf

Serves: 4
Preparation Time: 5 minutes
Cooking Time: 15 minutes
Ingredients
- 2 rice cups, rinsed
- 2 ½ cups, chicken stock
- 1 tablespoon rice wine
- 1 tablespoon vegetable oil
- 1 cup leftover chicken meat
- 2 small potatoes, peeled and quartered
- 2 carrots, chopped
- 1-pound white mushrooms, halved
- 1-pound green beans, chopped
- 3 cups kale, chopped
- 2 tablespoons soy sauce
- 1 tablespoon oyster sauce

Instructions
1. Place everything in the pot and give a good stir.
2. Give a good stir and close the lid.
3. Seal off the vent.
4. Press the Rice button and adjust the cooking time to 15 minutes.
5. Do natural pressure release.
6. Fluff the rice before serving.
Nutrition information:
Calories per serving: 506; Carbohydrates: 92.8g; Protein: 24.1g; Fat: 5.4g; Fiber: 8.6g

Instant Pot Ground Beef Shawarma Rice

Serves: 5
Preparation Time:5 minutes
Cooking Time: 15 minutes
Ingredients
- 1 tablespoon oil
- 1 cup onion, chopped
- 5 cloves of garlic, minced
- 1-pound ground beef
- 1 ½ cups water
- 1 ½ cups basmati rice, rinsed and drained
- 4 cups cabbage, shredded
- 3 tablespoons shawarma spice
- 1 teaspoon salt
- ¼ cup cilantro, chopped

Instructions
1. Place all ingredients in the Instant Pot except for the cilantro.
2. Give a good stir and close the lid.
3. Press the Manual button and adjust the cooking time to 15 minutes.
4. Do natural pressure release.
5. Once the lid is open, stir in the cilantro.
Nutrition information:
Calories per serving: 298; Carbohydrates: 30g; Protein: 12g; Fat: 13g; Fiber: 1g

Instant Pot Cajun Chicken and Rice

Serves: 5
Preparation Time: 10 minutes
Cooking Time:20 minutes
Ingredients
- 1 tablespoon oil
- 1 onion, diced
- 3 cloves of garlic, minced
- 1-pound chicken breasts, sliced
- 1 tablespoon Cajun seasoning
- 1 tablespoon tomato paste
- 2 cups chicken broth
- 1 ½ cups white rice, rinsed
- 1 bell pepper, chopped

Instructions
1. Press the Sauté on the Instant Pot and pour the oil.
2. Sauté the onion and garlic until fragrant.
3. Stir in the chicken breasts and season with Cajun seasoning.
4. Continue cooking for 3 minutes.
5. Add the tomato paste and chicken broth. Dissolve the tomato paste before adding the rice and bell pepper.
6. Close the lid and press the Manual button.
7. Adjust the cooking time to 20 minutes.
8. Do natural pressure release.
Nutrition information:
Calories per serving:473; Carbohydrates: 64.9g; Protein: 33.4g; Fat: 7.4g; Fiber: 2.9g

Hibachi Fried Rice

Serves: 6
Preparation Time: 5 minutes
Cooking Time: 15 minutes
Ingredients
- 2 cups Jasmine rice, rinsed and drained
- 2 cups water
- 1 tablespoon butter
- 3 eggs, beaten
- 1 onion, chopped
- 1 cup frozen peas
- 1 cup corn kernels
- 2 tablespoons soy sauce
- 2 tablespoons sesame oil

Instructions
1. Place the rice and water in the Instant Pot.
2. Close the lid and press the Manual button. Adjust the cooking time for 3 minutes.
3. Do natural pressure release to open the lid.
4. Fluff the rice and transfer to a serving bowl.
5. Press the Sauté button.
6. Use the same inner pot and melt the butter.
7. Scramble the eggs for a minute or two then set aside in a bowl.
8. Add the onions, peas, and corn.
9. Stir in the cooked rice and drizzle with soy sauce.
10. Add the scrambled eggs and continue stirring until the vegetables are cooked.
11. Drizzle with sesame oil last.
Nutrition information:
Calories per serving: 298; Carbohydrates: 28.9g; Protein: 11.6g; Fat: 20.9g; Fiber: 10.1g

Instant Pot Mexican Rice

Serves: 12
Preparation Time: 3 minutes
Cooking Time: 8 minutes

Ingredients
- 2 tablespoons olive oil
- ¼ cup onion, chopped
- 4 cloves of garlic, chopped
- 2 cups long grain white rice, rinsed
- A dash of salt
- ¾ cup crushed tomatoes
- 2 ½ cups chicken stock
- ½ teaspoon cumin
- ½ teaspoon smoked paprika
- ¼ cup sun-dried tomatoes

Instructions
1. Press the Sauté button on the Instant Pot.
2. Pour in the oil and sauté the onion and garlic until fragrant.
3. Add the rest of the ingredients and stir to combine everything.
4. Close the lid and press the Manual button.
5. Adjust the cooking time to 8 minutes.
6. Do natural pressure release.

Nutrition information:
Calories per serving: 158; Carbohydrates: 28.1g; Protein: 3.8g; Fat:3.5g; Fiber: 0.8g

Instant Pot Creamy Mushroom Wild Rice Soup

Serves: 6
Preparation Time: 5 minutes
Cooking Time: 45 minutes

Ingredients
- 5 carrots, chopped
- 5 stalks of celery, chopped
- 1 onion, chopped
- 3 cloves of garlic, minced
- 1 cup uncooked wild rice, rinsed
- 8 ounces mushrooms, diced
- 4 cups chicken broth
- 1 teaspoon salt
- 1 teaspoon dried thyme
- 6 tablespoons butter
- ½ cup flour
- 1 ½ cups milk

Instructions
1. Put all ingredients in the Instant Pot except the butter, flour, and milk.
2. Close the lid and press the Manual button. Adjust the cooking time to 45 minutes.
3. Meanwhile, prepare the sauce by melting the butter in a saucepan over medium flame. Whisk in the flour and add the milk gradually. Continue stirring until the sauce thickens.
4. Once the Instant Pot timer beeps, do natural pressure release. Fluff the rice and pour the creamy sauce. Stir to combine.

Nutrition information:
Calories per serving:670; Carbohydrates: 68.1g; Protein: 46.2g; Fat: 25.2g; Fiber:8.3g

Rice with Chicken and Broccoli

Serves: 6
Preparation Time: 5 minutes
Cooking Time: 15 minutes

Ingredients
- 2 tablespoons butter
- 1 ½ pounds boneless chicken breasts, sliced
- 2 cloves of garlic, minced
- 1 onion, chopped
- Salt and pepper to taste
- 1 1/3 cups long grain rice
- 1 1/3 cups chicken broth
- ½ cup milk
- 1 cup broccoli florets
- ½ cup cheddar cheese, grated

Instructions
1. Press the Sauté button on the Instant Pot.
2. Melt the butter and add the chicken pieces, garlic, and onion. Season with salt and pepper to taste.
3. Continue stirring for 5 minutes or until the chicken has slightly browned
4. Add the rice and chicken broth. Stir in the milk.
5. Stir in the broccoli florets and cheddar cheese.
6. Close the lid and seal off the vent.
7. Cook for15 minutes.
8. Do natural pressure release.

Nutrition information:
Calories per serving: 515; Carbohydrates: 41.6g; Protein: 47.9g; Fat: 16.6g; Fiber: 2.1g

Instant Pot Mushroom Risotto

Serves: 6
Preparation Time: 5 minutes
Cooking Time: 10 minutes

Ingredients
- 3 tablespoons olive oil
- 4 tablespoons unsalted butter
- 1 onion, chopped
- 4 cloves of garlic, minced
- 3 shiitake mushrooms, sliced
- 1 cremini mushrooms, sliced
- 2 cups Arborio rice
- 4 ½ cups chicken stock
- 1 cup parmesan cheese, grated
- 3 tablespoons light soy sauce
- ¾ cup dry white wine
- Salt and pepper to taste

Instructions
1. Press the Sauté button on the Instant Pot.
2. Heat the oil and butter.
3. Sauté the onion and garlic until fragrant.
4. Add the mushrooms.
5. Stir in the Arborio rice and half of the chicken stock.
6. Stir until the stock has boiled.
7. Add the rest of the ingredients and give a boil.
8. Close the lid and seal off the vent.
9. Press the Manual button and adjust the cooking time to 3 minutes.
10. Do natural pressure release.
11. Once the lid is open, press the Sauté button and continue stirring until the amount of liquid has reduced and the rice has thickened.

Nutrition information:

Calories per serving: 459; Carbohydrates: 60g; Protein: 11g; Fat:16 g; Fiber: 3g

Basic Instant Pot Risotto

Serves: 6
Preparation Time: 2 minutes
Cooking Time: 5 minutes

Ingredients
- 2 cups Arborio rice
- 4 cups chicken broth
- 1 onion, chopped
- 1 swig of white wine
- 1 tablespoon parmesan cheese, grated
- Salt and pepper to taste

Instructions
1. Press the Sauté button on the Instant Pot.
2. Place the rice, half of the chicken broth, onion, and wine.
3. Allow simmering for 3 minutes.
4. The rice should turn from solid white to translucent.
5. Pour the rest of the chicken broth and stir in the parmesan cheese. Season with salt and pepper to taste.
6. Close the lid.
7. Press the Manual button and adjust the cooking time to 4 minutes.
8. Do natural pressure release.
9. Press the Sauté button and allow to simmer until the right thickness.

Nutrition information:
Calories per serving: 393; Carbohydrates: 23.7g; Protein: 40.6g; Fat:19.5 g; Fiber: 8.1g

Instant Pot Porcini Risotto

Serves: 6
Preparation Time: 5 minutes
Cooking Time: 10 minutes

Ingredients
- 1 tablespoon olive oil
- ½ cup onions, chopped
- 1-ounce porcini mushrooms, sliced
- 1 ½ cups Arborio rice
- ½ cup dry white wine
- 3 ½ cups chicken broth
- Salt and pepper to taste
- 1 cup frozen peas
- ½ cup parmesan cheese

Instructions
1. Press the Sauté button on the Instant Pot.
2. Pour the oil and sauté the onions until fragrant. Stir in the mushrooms and cook for 2 minutes.
3. Add the rice, white wine and half of the chicken broth. Season with salt and pepper to taste.
4. Allow simmering for 3 minutes.
5. The rice should turn from solid white to translucent.
6. Pour the rest of the chicken broth.
7. Close the lid and press the Manual button and adjust the cooking time to 4 minutes.
8. Do natural pressure release.
9. Press the Sauté button and stir in the peas and parmesan cheese. Allow to cook for 5 minutes.

Nutrition information:
Calories per serving: 427; Carbohydrates: 23.6g; Protein: 39.9g; Fat: 22.5g; Fiber: 7.8g

Risotto with Bacon and Peas

Serves: 4
Preparation Time: 5 minutes
Cooking Time: 10 minutes

Ingredients
- 4 slices of bacon, chopped
- 2 tablespoons olive oil
- 1 onion, chopped
- 1 ½ cup Arborio rice
- ½ cup dry white wine
- 3 cups chicken broth
- Salt and pepper to taste
- 1 cup frozen peas
- ½ teaspoon lemon zest
- ½ cup parmesan cheese
- 3 tablespoons parsley

Instructions
1. Press the Sauté button on the Instant Pot.
2. Add the bacon. Allow the bacon to render. Set aside.
3. Pour olive oil and sauté the onion until fragrant.
4. Add the rice and stir for 30 seconds. Pour in the dry white wine and simmer until the wine has almost evaporated.
5. Pour in the chicken broth and season with salt and pepper to taste.
6. Close the lid and seal off the vent.
7. Press the Manual button and adjust the cooking time to4 minutes.
8. Do quick pressure release.
9. Once the lid is open, press the Sauté button and add the frozen peas and lemon zest.
10. Allow simmering without the lid on for 3 minutes.
11. Sprinkle with parmesan cheese, parsley, and bacon bits.

Nutrition information:
Calories per serving: 713; Carbohydrates: 32.2g; Protein: 56.2g; Fat: 42.5g; Fiber: 11.1g

Instant Pot Asparagus Risotto

Serves: 5
Preparation Time: 5 minutes
Cooking Time: 6 minutes

Ingredients
- 1 tablespoons olive oil
- 1 shallot, chopped
- 1 clove of garlic, minced
- 1 ½ cup Arborio rice
- 1/3 cup white wine
- 3 cups vegetable broth
- 1 teaspoon lemon zest
- 2 teaspoon thyme leaves
- Salt and pepper to taste
- 1 bunch asparagus spears, trimmed
- 1 tablespoons butter
- 2 tablespoons parmesan cheese, grated

Instructions
1. Press the Sauté button on the Instant Pot.
2. Pour the olive oil and sauté the shallot and garlic until fragrant

3. Add in the Arborio rice and stir for 30 seconds before adding the white wine.
4. Pour in the vegetable broth. Season with salt and pepper to taste.
5. Stir in the lemon zest and thyme leaves.
6. Close the lid and seal off the vent.
7. Press the Manual button and adjust the cooking time to 4 minutes.
8. Do quick pressure release.
9. Once the lid is open, press the Sauté button.
10. Stir in the asparagus spears and allow to simmer for 3 minutes.
11. Add the butter and sprinkle with parmesan cheese.
Nutrition information:
Calories per serving: 179; Carbohydrates: 21.4g; Protein:5.7g; Fat: 12.9g; Fiber: 7.7g

Butternut Squash Risotto

Serves: 6
Preparation Time: 5 minutes
Cooking Time: 10 minutes
Ingredients
- 2 tablespoons butter
- 3 cloves of garlic, minced
- 1 onion, chopped
- 3 tablespoons fresh sage, chopped
- 2 cups butternut squash, peeled and cubed
- 1 ½ cups Arborio rice
- 1.4 cup white wine
- 2 cups water
- 2 cups chicken stock
- Salt and pepper to taste
- 1 cup goat cheese, grated

Instructions
1. Press the Sauté button on the Instant Pot and melt butter.
2. Sauté the garlic, onions, and sage until fragrant.
3. Add in the butternut squash and sauté for 5 minutes.
4. Add the Arborio rice and white wine.
5. Allow simmering for 3 minutes until the wine has reduced.
6. Pour in water and chicken stock.
7. Season with salt and pepper to taste.
8. Close the lid and press the Manual button.
9. Adjust the cooking time to 4 minutes.
10. Do quick pressure release.
11. Once the lid is open, sprinkle with goat cheese.
Nutrition information:
Calories per serving: 205; Carbohydrates: 27.1g; Protein: 7.9g; Fat: 11.9g; Fiber: 8g

Spinach and Goat Cheese Risotto

Serves: 8
Preparation Time:10 minutes
Cooking Time: 10 minutes
Ingredients
- 2 tablespoons olive oil
- ¾ cup onion, chopped
- 2 cloves of garlic, minced
- 1 ½ cups Arborio rice
- ½ cup white wine
- 3 ½ cup hot vegetable broth
- Salt and pepper to taste
- 2 tablespoons lemon juice, freshly squeezed
- 1 cup spinach leaves, chopped
- ½ cup parmesan cheese, grated

Instructions
1. Press the Sauté button on the Instant Pot.
2. Pour the olive oil and sauté the onions and garlic until fragrant.
3. Add the Arborio rice and white wine.
4. Allow simmering for a minute before pouring in the hot vegetable broth.
5. Season with salt and pepper to taste
6. Close the lid and seal off the vent.
7. Press the Manual button and adjust the cooking time to 3 minutes.
8. Do quick pressure release.
9. Once the lid is open, press the Sauté button.
10. Add the lemon juice and spinach. Give a good stir and allow the spinach to wilt.
11. Sprinkle with parmesan cheese on top.
Nutrition information:
Calories per serving:146; Carbohydrates: 16.2g; Protein: 5.8g; Fat: 9.9g; Fiber: 5.5g

Roasted Cauliflower Barley Risotto

Serves: 4
Preparation Time: 5 minutes
Cooking Time: 25 minutes
Ingredients
- 1 head cauliflower, cut into florets
- 3 tablespoons olive oil
- 1 onion, chopped
- 2 cloves of garlic, minced
- 1 cup pearl barley, rinsed
- 3 cups vegetable broth
- Salt and pepper to taste
- 1 tablespoon butter
- ½ cup parmesan cheese, grated

Instructions
1. Press the Sauté button on the Instant Pot.
2. Pour the olive oil and sauté the onions and garlic until fragrant.
3. Add in the pearl barley and vegetable broth. Give a good stir.
4. Season with salt and pepper to taste.
5. Close the lid and seal off the vent.
6. Press the Manual button and adjust the cooking time to 20 minutes.
7. Do quick pressure release.
8. Once the lid is open, stir in the butter and sprinkle with parmesan cheese.
Nutrition information:
Calories per serving: 387; Carbohydrates: 50.8g; Protein:10.4g; Fat: 17.3g; Fiber: 9.8g

Instant Pot Pearl Barley

Serves: 5
Preparation Time: 2 minutes
Cooking Time: 25 minutes
Ingredients
- 1 ½ cups pearl barley
- 3 cups chicken broth

- 1 teaspoon salt

Instructions
1. Rinse and drain the barley.
2. Pour all ingredients into the Instant Pot. Give a good stir.
3. Close the lid and seal off the vent.
4. Press the Manual button and adjust the cooking time to 25 minutes.
5. Do natural pressure release.

Nutrition information:
Calories per serving: 439; Carbohydrates: 47.7g; Protein:37.1g; Fat: 10.7g; Fiber:9.3g

Pearl Barley Soup

Serves: 4
Preparation Time: 5 minutes
Cooking Time: 15 minutes

Ingredients
- 1 onion, chopped
- 1 carrot, chopped
- 1 leek, sliced
- 1 zucchini, sliced
- ½ butternut squash, diced
- ¾ cup pearl barley, soaked and rinsed
- 2 tablespoons tomato paste
- 7 cups chicken broth
- 1 teaspoon cumin
- 1 teaspoon paprika
- ½ teaspoon parsley
- Salt and pepper to taste

Instructions
1. Place all ingredients in the Instant Pot.
2. Give a good stir.
3. Close the lid and seal off the vent.
4. Press the Manual button and adjust the cooking time to 20 minutes.
5. Do quick pressure release.

Nutrition information:
Calories per serving:181; Carbohydrates:38.7 g; Protein: 8.3g; Fat: 0.4g; Fiber: 8.5g

Chicken Barley Soup

Serves: 6
Preparation Time: 5 minutes
Cooking Time: 20 minutes

Ingredients
- 3 cups chicken stock
- 2 cups water
- 2 cups carrots, diced
- 1 cup red potatoes, peeled and diced
- 1 cup onion, diced
- ¾ cup celery
- ½ cup pearl barley, rinsed and drained
- 1 tablespoon oregano
- 1 bay leaf
- 2 cups chicken breasts, sliced
- Salt and pepper to taste

Instructions
1. Place all ingredients in the Instant Pot.
2. Give a good stir.
3. Close the lid and seal off the vent.
4. Press the Manual button and adjust the cooking time to 20 minutes.
5. Do quick pressure release.

Nutrition information:
Calories per serving:313; Carbohydrates: 27.8g; Protein: 26.1g; Fat: 10.8g; Fiber: 4.7g

Beef Barley Soup

Serves: 6
Preparation Time: 10 minutes
Cooking Time: 30 minutes

Ingredients
- 2 tablespoons olive oil
- 4 cloves of garlic, minced
- 2 onions, chopped
- 1 stalk of celery, chopped
- 4 large carrots, chopped
- 2 pounds beef chuck roast
- 1 bay leaf
- 1 cup pearl barley, rinsed
- 1 tablespoon fish sauce
- Salt and pepper to taste

Instructions
1. Press the Sauté button on the Instant Pot.
2. Heat the oil and sauté the garlic, onions, and celery.
3. Add the carrots and beef chuck roast.
4. Stir in the bay leaf and pearl barley.
5. Season with fish sauce, salt, and pepper.
6. Close the lid.
7. Press the Manual button and adjust the cooking time to 30 minutes.
8. Do natural pressure release.

Nutrition information:
Calories per serving:476; Carbohydrates: 35.8g; Protein: 44.9g; Fat: 17.8g; Fiber:7.4g

Beefy Instant Pot Congee

Serves: 4
Preparation Time: 2 minutes
Cooking Time: 1 hour

Ingredients
- ½ pounds ground beef
- ¾ cup Jasmine rice, rinsed
- 7 cups cold water
- Salt to taste
- 1 green onion, chopped

Instructions
1. Place the ground beef, rice, and water in the Instant Pot.
2. Season with salt to taste.
3. Close the lid and press the Manual button.
4. Adjust the cooking time to 60 minutes.
5. Do natural pressure release.
6. Once the lid is off, add the green onion.
7. Adjust the seasoning if needed.

Nutrition information:
Calories per serving:219; Carbohydrates: 12.1g; Protein: 17.4g; Fat: 13.8g; Fiber: 5g

Vietnamese Chicken Congee (Chao Ga)

Serves: 6
Preparation Time: 2 minutes
Cooking Time: 1 hour

Ingredients
- 3 cups short-grain rice

- 2 pounds chicken thighs, skin and bones removed, sliced
- 4 quarts chicken broth
- 1 thumb-size ginger, minced
- 2 tablespoons soy sauce
- 2 tablespoons fish sauce
- 2 cups Thai basil

Instructions
1. Place all ingredients in the Instant Pot.
2. Close the lid and press the Manual button.
3. Adjust the cooking time to 60 minutes.
4. Do natural pressure release.
5. Garnish with cilantro or lime wedges.

Nutrition information:
Calories per serving: 719; Carbohydrates: 81.8g; Protein: 33.2g; Fat: 26.9g; Fiber: 2.9g

Instant Pot Basic Congee (Jook)

Serves: 6
Preparation Time: 10 minutes
Cooking Time: 1 hour

Ingredients
- 1 cup uncooked rice
- 2 cloves of garlic, minced
- 1 thumb-size ginger, minced
- 3 shiitake mushrooms, sliced
- 2 pounds chicken breasts, bone remove and sliced
- 7 cups water
- ½ tablespoon salt

Instructions
1. Place all ingredients in the Instant Pot.
2. Close the lid and press the Manual button.
3. Adjust the cooking time to 60 minutes.
4. Do natural pressure release.

Nutrition information:
Calories per serving: 329; Carbohydrates: 11.4g; Protein: 34.4g; Fat: 18.1g; Fiber: 4.3g

Brown Rice Congee with Shiitake Mushrooms

Serves: 4
Preparation Time: 2 minutes
Cooking Time: 1 hour

Ingredients
- ½ cup brown rice
- 4 cups mushroom broth
- 2 cup shiitake mushrooms, sliced
- 2 tablespoons minced ginger
- 2 cloves of garlic, minced
- 3 cups warm water
- Salt to taste

Instructions
1. Place all ingredients in the Instant Pot.
2. Close the lid and press the Manual button.
3. Adjust the cooking time to 60 minutes.
4. Do natural pressure release.

Nutrition information:
Calories per serving: 178; Carbohydrates: 29.6g; Protein: 5.2g; Fat: 4.7g; Fiber: 1.3g

Festive Chicken Ginger Congee

Serves: 8
Preparation Time: 2 minutes
Cooking Time: 40 minutes

Ingredients
- 8 cups water
- 3 boneless chicken thighs, sliced
- 1 cup long-grain rice, rinsed
- 4 thick slices of ginger, smashed
- 2 teaspoons salt
- ½ cup roasted peanuts
- ½ cup scallions, chopped
- 3 tablespoons ginger, minced
- ½ cup cilantro leaves

Instructions
1. Place the first 5 ingredients in the Instant Pot.
2. Close the lid and seal off the vent.
3. Press the Manual button and adjust the cooking time to 40 minutes.
4. Do natural pressure release.
5. Before serving, sprinkle with the remaining ingredients on top.

Nutrition information:
Calories per serving: 351; Carbohydrates: 32.4g; Protein: 16g; Fat: 18g; Fiber: 2g

Instant Pot Buckwheat Porridge

Serves: 4
Preparation Time: 2 minutes
Cooking Time: 6 minutes

Ingredients
- 1 cup buckwheat groats
- 3 cups milk
- 1 banana, sliced
- ¼ cup raisins
- 1 teaspoon ground cinnamon
- ½ teaspoon vanilla
- Chopped nuts for garnish

Instructions
1. Place all ingredients except the nuts in the Instant Pot.
2. Close the lid and seal off the vent.
3. Press the Manual button and adjust the cooking time to 6 minutes.
4. Do natural pressure release.
5. Sprinkle with nuts on top.

Nutrition information:
Calories per serving: 322; Carbohydrates: 39.8g; Protein: 18.4g; Fat: 11.1g; Fiber: 4g

Basic Instant Pot Quinoa

Serves: 6
Preparation Time: 2 minutes
Cooking Time: 12 minutes

Ingredients
- 1 cup quinoa, rinsed
- 2 cups water

Instructions
1. Place all ingredients in the Instant Pot.
2. Close the lid and seal off the vent.
3. Press the Manual button and adjust the cooking time to 12 minutes.
4. Do natural pressure release.

Nutrition information:
Calories per serving: 104; Carbohydrates: 18.18g; Protein: 4g; Fat: 1.72g; Fiber: 2g

One-Minute Quinoa and Veggies

Serves: 4
Preparation Time: 2 minutes
Cooking Time: 2 minutes
Ingredients
- 3 stalks of celery, chopped
- 1 bell pepper, chopped
- 1 ½ cups quinoa, rinsed
- ¼ teaspoon salt
- 4 cups spinach
- 1 ½ cups chicken broth
- ½ cup feta cheese

Instructions
1. Place all ingredients except the feta cheese in the Instant Pot.
2. Close the lid and seal off the vent.
3. Press the Manual button and adjust the cooking time to 2 minutes.
4. Do natural pressure release.
5. Once the lid is open, garnish with feta cheese on top.

Nutrition information:
Calories per serving: 360; Carbohydrates: 31g; Protein: 16g; Fat: 18g; Fiber: 9g

Mexican Quinoa with Cilantro Sauce

Serves: 4
Preparation Time: 5 minutes
Cooking Time: 10 minutes
Ingredients
- 2 tablespoons cilantro, chopped
- ½ clove of garlic, minced
- 1 tablespoon lime juice
- 2 tablespoons mayonnaise
- 1 tablespoons jalapeno, chopped
- A pinch of salt
- 2 tablespoons olive oil
- 1 onion, chopped
- 3 cloves of garlic, minced
- 1 red pepper, diced
- 1 stalk of celery, diced
- 1 teaspoon cumin
- 1 teaspoon coriander seeds
- 1 teaspoon paprika
- 1 teaspoon oregano
- 1 cup raw quinoa, rinsed
- Salt and pepper to taste
- ½ cup corn kernels
- ½ cup garden peas
- ½ cup tomato puree
- ½ cup water

Instructions
1. Prepare the cilantro sauce first by combining in a small bowl the first 5 ingredients. Set aside.
2. Press the Sauté button on the Instant Pot.
3. Heat the oil and sauté the onion and garlic until fragrant.
4. Add the pepper and celery. Season with cumin, coriander, paprika, and oregano.
5. Stir in the quinoa and season with salt and pepper to taste.
6. Dump the corn, peas, tomato puree, and water.
7. Close the lid and seal off the vent.
8. Press the Manual button and adjust the cooking time to 12 minutes.
9. Do natural pressure release.
10. Serve with cilantro sauce.

Nutrition information:
Calories per serving: 298; Carbohydrates: 40.3g; Protein: 8.7g; Fat: 12.3g; Fiber: 5.6g

Quinoa Fried Rice

Serves: 6
Preparation Time: 5 minutes
Cooking Time: 20 minutes
Ingredients
- 3 ½ cups quinoa, rinsed
- 3 cups water
- 1 tablespoon sesame oil
- 3 cloves of garlic, minced
- 1 onion, diced
- 1 cup frozen mixed vegetables
- 2 large eggs, beaten
- 2 tablespoons soy sauce
- 1 teaspoon red pepper flakes
- Salt and pepper to taste

Instructions
1. Place the quinoa and water in the Instant Pot.
2. Close the lid and press the Manual button. Adjust the cooking time to 12 minutes.
3. Do natural pressure release. Take the cooked quinoa out and set aside in another bowl.
4. Press the Sauté button on the pot.
5. Heat the sesame oil and sauté the garlic and onion until fragrant.
6. Add the vegetables and stir for 3 minutes. Push the vegetables to one side and add the eggs.
7. Scramble the eggs.
8. Stir in the cooked quinoa and season with soy sauce, red pepper flakes, salt, and pepper.
9. Stir to combine everything.
10. Serve warm.

Nutrition information:
Calories per serving: 454; Carbohydrates: 72.7g; Protein: 16.7g; Fat: 10.8g; Fiber: 9g

Instant Pot Quinoa Pilaf

Serves: 6
Preparation Time: 10 minutes
Cooking Time: 20 minutes
Ingredients
- 3 tablespoons butter
- 2 tablespoons onion, chopped
- 1 tablespoon garlic, minced
- 2 tablespoons chopped celery
- 2 cups quinoa, rinsed
- 2 cups chicken broth
- ¾ teaspoon garlic powder
- ¼ teaspoon paprika
- Salt and pepper to taste
- 1 tablespoon parsley, chopped

Instructions
1. Press the Sauté button on the Instant Pot.
2. Melt the butter and sauté the onion, garlic, and celery until fragrant.

3. Add the quinoa, chicken broth, garlic, powder, and paprika.
4. Season with salt and pepper to taste.
5. Close the lid and press the Manual button.
6. Adjust the cooking time to 15 minutes
7. Do natural pressure release.
8. Garnish with parsley on top
Nutrition information:
Calories per serving:592; Carbohydrates: 58.4g; Protein: 38.6g; Fat: 22.2g; Fiber: 6.4g

Quinoa with Mushrooms and Vegetables

Serves: 6
Preparation Time: 2 minutes
Cooking Time: 12 minutes
Ingredients
- 3 tablespoons olive oil
- 1 onion, diced
- 1 carrots, peeled and chopped
- 2 cups button mushrooms, sliced
- Zest of ½ lemon
- 2 tablespoons lemon juice
- 1 tablespoon salt
- 4 cloves of garlic, minced
- 1 cup quinoa, rinsed
- 1 cup vegetable stock

Instructions
1. Place all ingredients in the Instant Pot.
2. Close the lid and press the Manual button.
3. Adjust the cooking time to 12 minutes.
4. Do natural pressure release.

Nutrition information:
Calories per serving: 184; Carbohydrates: 22.2g; Protein: 4.5g; Fat: 8.5; Fiber: 4.3g

Basic Instant Pot Millet

Serves: 4
Preparation Time: 2 minutes
Cooking Time: 9 minutes
Ingredients
- ½ cup millet
- 1 cup water

Instructions
1. Place all ingredients in the Instant Pot.
2. Close the lid and press the Manual button.
3. Adjust the cooking time to 9 minutes.

Nutrition information:
Calories per serving: 95; Carbohydrates: 18.2g; Protein: 2.8g; Fat: 1.1g; Fiber:2.1g

Instant Pot Millet Porridge

Serves: 3
Preparation Time: 5 minutes
Cooking Time: 10 minutes
Ingredients
- 3 tablespoons of prepared millet
- 1 ½ cups coconut milk
- 2 Medjool dates, chopped
- 1 teaspoon cinnamon powder
- 1 teaspoon vanilla powder
- A dash of salt

Instructions
1. Place all ingredients in the Instant Pot.
2. Close the lid and press the Manual button.
3. Adjust the cooking time to 10 minutes.

Nutrition information:
Calories per serving:374; Carbohydrates: 28.6g; Protein: 4.5g; Fat: 29.7g; Fiber: 5.1g

Creamy Millet Breakfast Porridge

Serves: 2
Preparation Time: 5 minutes
Cooking Time:20 minutes
Ingredients
- 1 cup uncooked millet
- 1 cup almond milk
- 3 cups water
- 2 tablespoons maple syrup
- 1 tablespoon vanilla extract
- Chopped almonds, for garnish
- Sliced strawberries, for garnish

Instructions
1. Place all ingredients except for the almonds and strawberries in the Instant Pot.
2. Close the lid and press the Manual button.
3. Adjust the cooking time to 20 minutes.

Nutrition information:
Calories per serving:514; Carbohydrates: 98.9g; Protein: 11.9g; Fat: 6.5g; Fiber: 9.2g

Proofing Whole Wheat Bread in Instant Pot

Serves: 6
Preparation Time: 4 hours
Cooking Time: 30 minutes
Ingredients
- 2 ¼ cups whole wheat flour
- 1 cup white flour
- 2 tablespoons vital wheat gluten
- 2 tablespoons rolled oats
- 1 tablespoon raw millet
- 1 tablespoon flax seeds
- 1 tablespoon sunflower seeds
- 1 ½ teaspoon salt
- 1 teaspoon instant yeast
- 1 ½ cups water, room temperature

Instructions
1. In a bowl, mix together the wheat flour, white flour, gluten, oats, millet, flax seed, sunflower seeds, salt, and yeast.
2. Add water gradually and mix until the dough becomes tacky but not too overly wet.
3. Place on top of a parchment paper and place inside the Instant Pot.
4. Close the lid without sealing the vent.
5. Press the Yogurt button. Adjust the screen until it reads 24:00. Set the pressure to low.
6. Adjust the time to 4:30 and once the timer beeps off after 4 hours, the bread should have proofed.
7. Form a ball and place back on the parchment paper.
8. Heat the oven to 450 degrees Fahrenheit.
9. Place the bread in the oven and cook for 30 minutes.

Nutrition information:

Calories per serving: 261; Carbohydrates: 51.9g; Protein: 9.5g; Fat: 3.1g; Fiber: 6.2g

Instant Pot Coconut Oatmeal

Serves: 2
Preparation Time: 2 minutes
Cooking Time: 3 minutes

Ingredients
- 1 cup steel-cut oats
- 2 cups water
- 1 cup coconut milk
- ½ cup coconut sugar
- 1 apple, cored and sliced

Instructions
1. Place all ingredients in the Instant Pot.
2. Stir to combine.
3. Close the lid and press the Manual button.
4. Adjust the cooking time to 3 minutes.
5. Do natural pressure release.

Nutrition information:
Calories per serving: 536; Carbohydrates: 75.3g; Protein: 11.1g; Fat: 32.1g; Fiber: 12.1g

Banana Walnut Steel-Cut Oats

Serves: 3
Preparation Time: 2 minutes
Cooking Time: 6 minutes

Ingredients
- 1 cup steel-cut oats
- 2 cups water
- 1 cup almond milk
- ¼ cup walnut, chopped
- 2 tablespoons flaxseed
- 2 tablespoons chia seeds
- 1 large banana, sliced
- 2 tablespoons pure maple syrup
- 1 teaspoon cinnamon powder
- 1 teaspoon pure vanilla extract
- A pinch of salt

Instructions
1. Place all ingredients in the Instant Pot.
2. Stir to combine.
3. Close the lid and press the Manual button.
4. Adjust the cooking time to 6 minutes.
5. Do natural pressure release.

Nutrition information:
Calories per serving: 295; Carbohydrates: 52.7g; Protein: 9.3g; Fat: 11.6g; Fiber: 10.3 g

Instant Pot Apple Spice Oats

Serves: 2
Preparation Time: 2 minutes
Cooking Time: 6 minutes

Ingredients
- ½ cup steel cut oats
- 1 medium apple, peeled and chopped
- 1 ½ cups water
- 1 teaspoon ground cinnamon
- ¼ teaspoon allspice
- 1/8 teaspoon nutmeg
- 3 tablespoons maple syrup

Instructions
1. Place all ingredients in the Instant Pot.
2. Stir to combine.
3. Close the lid and press the Manual button.
4. Adjust the cooking time to 6 minutes.
5. Do natural pressure release.

Nutrition information:
Calories per serving: 188; Carbohydrates: 49.5g; Protein: 4.4g; Fat: 1.9g; Fiber: 6.6g

Pumpkin Spice Oat Meal

Serves: 6
Preparation Time: 2 minutes
Cooking Time: 10 minutes

Ingredients
- 1 can pumpkin puree
- 1 ¼ cups steel-cut oats
- 3 tablespoons brown sugar
- 1 ½ teaspoons pumpkin pie spice
- 1 teaspoon ground cinnamon
- ¾ teaspoon salt
- 3 cups water
- 1 ½ cups milk

Instructions
1. Place all ingredients in the Instant Pot.
2. Stir to combine.
3. Close the lid and press the Manual button.
4. Adjust the cooking time to 10 minutes.
5. Do natural pressure release.

Nutrition information:
Calories per serving: 127; Carbohydrates: 26.g; Protein: 6.3g; Fat: 3.7g; Fiber: 5.7g

Peaches and Cream Oatmeal

Serves: 8
Preparation Time: 2 minutes
Cooking Time: 10 minutes

Ingredients
- 4 cups old-fashioned oats
- 3 ½ cups water
- 3 ½ cups milk
- 1 teaspoon salt
- 1 teaspoon ground cinnamon
- 1/3 cup sugar
- 4 peaches

Instructions
1. Place all ingredients in the Instant Pot.
2. Stir to combine.
3. Close the lid and press the Manual button.
4. Adjust the cooking time to 10 minutes.
5. Do natural pressure release.

Nutrition information:
Calories per serving: 222; Carbohydrates: 47.1g; Protein: 11.7g; Fat: 6.8g; Fiber: 7.8g

Chicken Recipes

Lemon Olive Chicken

Serves: 8
Preparation Time: 5 minutes
Cooking Time: 10 minutes
Ingredients
- 4 chicken breasts, bones, and skin removed
- ½ teaspoon cumin
- 1 teaspoon salt
- ½ teaspoon black pepper
- ½ cup butter, melted
- Juice of 1 lemon
- 1 cup chicken broth
- 1 can pitted green olives

Instructions
1. In a bowl, season the chicken breasts with cumin, salt, and pepper.
2. Press the Sauté button on the Instant Pot and place the chicken meat and butter.
3. Brown all sides for 3 minutes.
4. Add the rest of the ingredients.
5. Close the lid and press the Poultry button.
6. Adjust the cooking time for 10 minutes.
7. Do quick pressure release.

Nutrition information:
Calories per serving: 401; Carbohydrates: 0.8g; Protein: 36.9g; Fat: 27g; Fiber: 0.2g

Italian Chicken Marsala

Serves: 4
Preparation Time: 6 minutes
Cooking Time: 15 minutes
Ingredients
- 2 chicken breasts, bones, and skin removed
- Salt and pepper to taste
- ¼ cup potato starch
- 3 tablespoons olive oil
- 2 tablespoons butter
- 2 onions, chopped
- 3 cloves of garlic, minced
- 1-pound cremini mushrooms, sliced
- 1 cup dry marsala wine
- ½ teaspoon herbes de provence
- ½ cup chicken stock

Instructions
1. Season the chicken with salt and pepper. Dredge into potato starch. Set aside.
2. Press the Sauté button on the Instant Pot. Heat olive oil.
3. Place the dredged chicken pieces and allow to brown lightly for 3 minutes on each side. Set aside.
4. Place the butter and sauté the onions and garlic until fragrant.
5. Add the rest of the ingredients and place the chicken.
6. Season with more salt and pepper to taste.
7. Close the lid and press the Poultry button.
8. Adjust the cooking time to 15 minutes.
9. Do natural pressure release.

Nutrition information:
Calories per serving: 207; Carbohydrates: 25.5g; Protein: 11.6g; Fat: 8.3g; Fiber: 3.8g

Instant Pot Chicken Cacciatore

Serves: 4
Preparation Time: 5 minutes
Cooking Time: 20 minutes
Ingredients
- 4 chicken thighs, skin and bones removed
- Salt and pepper to taste
- ½ can crushed tomatoes
- ½ cup onion, diced
- ¼ cup red bell pepper, diced
- ½ cup green bell pepper, diced
- ½ teaspoon dried oregano
- 1 bay leaf

Instructions
1. Place all ingredients in the Instant Pot.
2. Give a good stir.
3. Close the lid and press the Poultry button.
4. Adjust the cooking time to 20 minutes.
5. Do natural pressure release.

Nutrition information:
Calories per serving: 133; Carbohydrates: 10.5g; Protein: 14g; Fat: 3g; Fiber: 1g

Honey Bourbon Chicken

Serves: 4
Preparation Time: 5 minutes
Cooking Time: 20 minutes
Ingredients
- 1 tablespoon oil
- 3 cloves of garlic, minced
- ½ cup onion, diced
- 1 ½ pounds chicken thighs, bones, and skin removed
- Salt and pepper
- ½ cup soy sauce
- ¼ cup ketchup
- ¼ teaspoon red pepper flakes
- 1 cup honey

Instructions
1. Press the Sauté button on the Instant Pot.
2. Pour the oil and sauté the garlic and onion until fragrant.
3. Stir in the chicken and season with salt, pepper, and soy sauce.
4. After 5 minutes, add the rest of the ingredients.
5. Close the lid and press the Poultry button.
6. Adjust the cooking time to 15 minutes.
7. Do natural pressure release.

Nutrition information:
Calories per serving: 786; Carbohydrates: 85.7g; Protein: 31.3g; Fat: 37.5g; Fiber: 1.4g

Butter Chicken Murgh Makhani

Serves: 4
Preparation Time: 3 minutes
Cooking Time: 20 minutes
Ingredients
- 1 can crushed tomatoes
- 6 cloves of garlic
- 2 teaspoons ginger, grated
- 1 teaspoon turmeric

- ½ teaspoon cayenne pepper
- 1 teaspoon paprika
- 1 teaspoon garam masala
- 1 teaspoon cumin
- 1-pound chicken meat

Instructions
1. Put everything in the Instant Pot.
2. Close the lid and press the Poultry button.
3. Adjust the cooking time to 20 minutes.
4. Do natural pressure release.

Nutrition information:
Calories per serving: 200; Carbohydrates: 4.5g; Protein: 23.9g; Fat:9.6g; Fiber:1.5g

Honey Sesame Chicken

Serves: 6
Preparation Time: 5 minutes
Cooking Time: 25 minutes

Ingredients
- 1 tablespoon oil
- ½ cup diced onions
- 2 cloves of garlic, minced
- 4 large chicken breasts, bones, and skin removed
- Salt and pepper
- ½ cup soy sauce
- ¼ cup ketchup
- 2 teaspoons sesame oil
- ½ cup honey
- ¼ teaspoon red pepper flakes
- 2 green onion, chopped
- 1 tablespoon sesame seeds, toasted

Instructions
1. Press the Sauté button on the Instant Pot.
2. Pour the oil and sauté the onions and garlic until fragrant.
3. Stir in the chicken meat and season with salt and pepper.
4. Cook for 3 minutes on each side.
5. Add the soy sauce, ketchup, sesame oil, honey, and red pepper flakes.
6. Close the lid and press the Poultry button.
7. Adjust the cooking time to 20 minutes.
8. Do natural pressure release.
9. Garnish with onions and sesame seeds.

Nutrition information:
Calories per serving:628; Carbohydrates: 34.9g; Protein: 64.1g; Fat: 25.3g; Fiber: 1.9g

Instant Pot Rotisserie Chicken

Serves: 6
Preparation Time: 5 minutes
Cooking Time: 40 minutes

Ingredients
- 1 whole chicken
- 1 ½ teaspoons salt
- ½ teaspoon pepper
- 1 teaspoon minced garlic
- 1 teaspoon paprika
- 1 ¾ tablespoons olive oil
- 1 cup chicken broth

Instructions
1. In a mixing bowl, mix all ingredients except for the chicken broth.
2. Make sure to massage the chicken until all surfaces are covered by the spice rub.
3. Pour the chicken broth into the Instant Pot.
4. Add the chicken.
5. Close the lid and press the Poultry button.
6. Adjust the cooking time to 40 minutes.
7. Do natural pressure release.

Nutrition information:
Calories per serving: 564; Carbohydrates: 45.8g; Protein:45.5 g; Fat: 22.6g; Fiber: 7g

Instant Pot Shredded Chicken

Serves: 8
Preparation Time: 3 minutes
Cooking Time: 30 minutes

Ingredients
- 4 pounds chicken breasts
- ½ cup water
- Salt and pepper to taste

Instructions
1. Place all ingredients in the Instant Pot.
2. Close the lid and press the Poultry button.
3. Adjust the cooking time to 30 minutes.
4. Do natural pressure release.
5. Use two forks to shred the chicken meat. Remove bones if any.

Nutrition information:
Calories per serving:392; Carbohydrates: 0.5g; Protein: 47.4g; Fat: 21g; Fiber: 0g

Instant Pot Mongolian Chicken

Serves: 6
Preparation Time: 5 minutes
Cooking Time: 15 minutes

Ingredients
- 2 tablespoons olive oil
- 1 onion, minced
- 10 cloves of garlic, minced
- chicken breasts, cut into cubes
- 1 tablespoon ginger, grated
- 1 cup brown sugar
- 1 cup soy sauce
- 1 cup water
- 1 cup carrots, chopped
- 1 teaspoons red pepper flakes
- 1 tablespoon garlic powder
- 2 tablespoons water + 1 tablespoon cornstarch

Instructions
1. Press the Sauté button on the Instant Pot.
2. Pour the oil and sauté the onions and garlic until fragrant.
3. Stir in the chicken meat and cook for 3 minutes on each side.
4. Place the remaining ingredients except for the cornstarch slurry in the Instant Pot.
5. Close the lid and press the Poultry button.
6. Adjust the cooking time to 15 minutes.
7. Do natural pressure release.
8. Once the lid is open, press the Sauté button.
9. Add the cornstarch slurry.
10. Simmer until thick.

Nutrition information:

Calories per serving:340; Carbohydrates: 39g; Protein: 20g; Fat: 6g; Fiber: 1g

Instant Pot Chicken Adobo

Serves: 4
Preparation Time: 3 minutes
Cooking Time: 30 minutes
Ingredients
- 4 chicken legs
- Salt and pepper to taste
- 1/3 cup soy sauce
- ¼ cup sugar
- ¼ cup white vinegar
- 2 bay leaves
- 5 cloves of garlic, crushed
- 1 onion, chopped

Instructions
1. Place all ingredients in the Instant Pot.
2. Close the lid and press the Poultry button.
3. Adjust the cooking time to 30 minutes.
4. Do natural pressure release.

Nutrition information:
Calories per serving:428; Carbohydrates: 16.8g; Protein: 53g; Fat:15.1g; Fiber: 1.1g

Moringa Chicken Soup

Serves: 8
Preparation Time: 3 minutes
Cooking Time: 15 minutes
Ingredients
- 1 ½ pounds chicken breasts
- Salt and pepper
- 2 cloves of garlic, minced
- 1 onion, chopped
- 5 cups water
- 1 thumb-size ginger
- 1 cup tomatoes, chopped
- 2 cups moringa leaves or kale leaves

Instructions
1. Place all ingredients in the Instant Pot except for the moringa leaves.
2. Close the lid and press the Poultry button.
3. Adjust the cooking time to 15 minutes.
4. Do natural pressure release.
5. Once the lid is open, press the Sauté button.
6. Stir in the moringa leaves and simmer for 3 minutes.

Nutrition information:
Calories per serving: 161; Carbohydrates: 3.6g; Protein: 18.5g; Fat:7.9 g; Fiber: 0.5g

Lemon Mustard Chicken with Potatoes

Serves: 8
Preparation Time: 6 minutes
Cooking Time: 15 minutes
Ingredients
- 2 tablespoons olive oil
- 2 pounds chicken thighs
- 3 tablespoons Dijon mustard
- 2 tablespoons Italian seasoning
- 3 pounds red potatoes, peeled and quartered
- ¾ cup chicken broth
- ¼ cup lemon juice
- Salt and pepper

Instructions
1. Press the Sauté button on the Instant Pot.
2. Pour the oil and place the chicken meat.
3. Cook until the chicken has turned light brown.
4. Add the Dijon mustard, Italian seasoning, and potatoes. Stir for 2 minutes.
5. Pour in the chicken broth and lemon juice. Season with salt and pepper to taste.
6. Scrape the bottom of the pot to remove the browning.
7. Close the lid and press the Poultry button.
8. Adjust the cooking time to 15 minutes.
9. Do natural pressure release.

Nutrition information:
Calories per serving:450; Carbohydrates: 30.7g; Protein: 27.4g; Fat: 24g; Fiber: 3.5g

Lemongrass and Coconut Chicken

Serves: 4
Preparation Time: 5 minutes
Cooking Time: 15 minutes
Ingredients
- 10 chicken drumsticks
- 1 onion, sliced
- 4 cloves of garlic, minced
- 1 stalk lemongrass, trimmed and cut to 2 inches thick
- 1 thumb-size ginger
- 2 tablespoons fish sauce
- 3 tablespoons soy sauce
- 1 teaspoon five spice powder
- 1 cup coconut milk
- ¼ cup cilantro, chopped
- Salt and pepper

Instructions
1. Press the Sauté button on the Instant Pot.
2. Place the chicken, onion, and garlic. Cook until the chicken has rendered some oil and turn slightly brown. Cook for 6 minutes.
3. Add the rest of the ingredients.
4. Close the lid and press the Poultry button.
5. Adjust the cooking time to 15 minutes.
6. Do natural pressure release.

Nutrition information:
Calories per serving: 711; Carbohydrates:9.8 g; Protein: 61.9g; Fat: 46.3g; Fiber: 2g

Instant Pot Crack Chicken

Serves: 8
Preparation Time: 3 minutes
Cooking Time: 15 minutes
Ingredients
- 2 pounds chicken breasts, bones removed
- 1 packet ranch seasoning
- 8 ounces cream cheese
- 1 cup water
- 4 ounces cheddar cheese, grated
- 6 slices of bacon, fried and crumbled

Instructions
1. Place the chicken in the Instant Pot.
2. Sprinkle with ranch seasoning.

3. Pour in the cream cheese, water, and cheddar cheese.
4. Close the lid and press the Poultry button.
5. Adjust the cooking time to 15 minutes.
6. Do natural pressure release.
7. Once the lid is open, sprinkle with crumbled bacon.

Nutrition information:
Calories per serving: 383; Carbohydrates: 2.7g; Protein: 30g; Fat: 27.5g; Fiber:0g

Instant Pot Chicken Biryani

Serves: 8
Preparation Time: 30 minutes
Cooking Time: 30 minutes

Ingredients
- 2 teaspoon garam masala
- 1 tablespoon ginger paste
- 1 tablespoon garlic paste
- ½ teaspoon turmeric
- 1 tablespoon red chili powder
- ¼ cup cilantro, chopped
- ¼ cup mint leaves
- ¾ cup yogurt
- 2 tablespoons lemon juice
- 2 pounds whole chicken, cut into 12 pieces
- 3 tablespoons ghee
- 2 onions, sliced
- 1 jalapeno, chopped
- 3 cups basmati rice, soaked then rinsed
- Salt
- 3 cups water
- 1 teaspoon saffron + 1 tablespoon milk
- 6 hard-boiled eggs, peeled

Instructions
1. Make the marinade by mixing in the bowl the garam masala, ginger paste, garlic paste, turmeric and red chili powder. Add the cilantro, mint, yogurt, and lemon juice. Marinate the chicken for at least 30 minutes in the fridge.
2. While the chicken is marinating, press the Sauté button on the Instant Pot. Add 1 tablespoon of the ghee and sauté the onions for 15 minutes until golden brown and caramelized. Set aside.
3. Use another tablespoon of ghee and sauté the jalapeno. Stir in the marinated chicken. Stir constantly for 3 minutes.
4. Close the lid and seal the vent. Press the Manual button and adjust the cooking time to 5 minutes. Do quick pressure release.
5. Once the lid is open, pour the rice over the chicken and add salt to taste and 3 cups of water. Stir in the saffron with milk.
6. Close the lid and press the Manual button. Adjust the cooking time to 8 minutes.
7. Do quick pressure release.
8. Fluff the rice with the chicken and garnish with eggs and cooked onions. Sprinkle with chopped cilantro if desired.

Nutrition information:
Calories per serving:471; Carbohydrates: 65.1g; Protein: 30.3; Fat: 8.9g; Fiber: 2.2g

Smokey Honey Cilantro Chicken

Serves: 10
Preparation Time: 3 minutes
Cooking Time: 15 minutes

Ingredients
- 1 cup salsa Verde
- ¼ cup honey
- 1 tablespoon liquid smoke
- 2 teaspoons chili powder
- 1 teaspoon dried oregano
- 1 teaspoon cumin
- ½ teaspoon smoked paprika
- 3 pounds chicken breasts, bones, and skin removed
- Salt and pepper
- ½ cup cilantro, chopped

Instructions
1. Place in the Instant Pot all ingredients except for the cilantro.
2. Stir to coat the chicken.
3. Close the lid and press the Manual button.
4. Adjust the cooking time to 15 minutes.
5. Do quick pressure release.
6. Once the lid is off, stir in cilantro.

Nutrition information:
Calories per serving: 274; Carbohydrates: 9.5g; Protein: 28.9g; Fat: 12.9g; Fiber: 0.9g

Thai Chicken Stew

Serves: 8
Preparation Time: 5 minutes
Cooking Time: 15 minutes

Ingredients
- 3 pounds chicken thighs
- 1 onion, sliced
- 2 cloves of garlic, minced
- 1 can coconut milk
- 1/3 cup tomato paste
- ½ cup Thai red curry paste
- 2 tablespoons fish sauce
- 2 tablespoons coconut aminos
- 2 teaspoons fresh lime juice
- ¾ teaspoon grated ginger
- 4 cups mixed vegetables
- Salt
- Fresh cilantro for garnish

Instructions
1. Press the Sauté button on the Instant Pot.
2. Add the chicken, onion, and garlic. Stir to turn the chicken golden on all sides.
3. Pour in the rest of the ingredients except for the cilantro.
4. Give a good stir.
5. Close the lid and press the Manual button.
6. Adjust the cooking time to 10 minutes.
7. Do quick pressure release.
8. Once the lid is open, stir in the cilantro.

Nutrition information:
Calories per serving: 538; Carbohydrates: 20.3g; Protein: 33.1g; Fat: 36.4g; Fiber: 8.5g

Chili Lime Chicken

Serves: 8
Preparation Time: 5 minutes

Cooking Time: 15 minutes
Ingredients
- 2 pounds chicken breasts, bones removed
- Juice of 2 medium limes
- 1 ½ teaspoons chili powder
- 1 teaspoon cumin
- 1 teaspoon onion powder
- 6 cloves garlic, minced
- ½ teaspoon liquid smoke
- Salt and pepper

Instructions
1. Place all ingredients in the Instant Pot.
2. Give a good stir.
3. Close the lid and press the Manual button.
4. Adjust the cooking time to 15 minutes.
5. Do quick pressure release.

Nutrition information:
Calories per serving: 207; Carbohydrates: 2.8g; Protein: 24.1g; Fat: 10.7g; Fiber: 0.5g

Honey Teriyaki Chicken

Serves: 8
Preparation Time: 3 minutes
Cooking Time: 15 minutes
Ingredients
- 8 chicken thighs
- ½ cup soy sauce
- ¼ cup rice vinegar
- 2 cloves of garlic, minced
- 2 teaspoons grated ginger
- 2 tablespoons honey
- ¼ teaspoon black pepper
- 1 tablespoon cornstarch + 2 tablespoons water
- 2 tablespoons sesame seeds, toasted
- 2 tablespoons chopped green onions

Instructions
1. Place all ingredients except for the cornstarch slurry, sesame seeds, and green onions in the Instant Pot.
2. Give a good stir.
3. Close the lid and press the Manual button.
4. Adjust the cooking time to 15 minutes.
5. Do quick pressure release.
6. Once the lid is open, press the Sauté button and stir in the slurry.
7. Allow simmering until the sauce thickens.
8. Stir in the sesame seeds and green onions last.

Nutrition information:
Calories per serving: 200; Carbohydrates: 9g; Protein: 22g; Fat: 9g; Fiber: 0g

Instant Pot Cashew Chicken

Serves: 6
Preparation Time: 3 minutes
Cooking Time: 15 minutes
Ingredients
- 2 pounds chicken thighs, bones, and skin removed
- ¼ teaspoon black pepper
- ¼ cup soy sauce
- 2 tablespoons rice vinegar
- 2 tablespoons ketchup
- 1 tablespoon brown sugar
- 1 clove of garlic, minced
- 1 teaspoon grated ginger
- 1 tablespoon cornstarch + 2 tablespoons water
- 1/3 cup cashew nuts, toasted
- ¼ cup green onions, chopped
- 2 tablespoons sesame seeds, toasted

Instructions
1. Place all ingredients except for the cornstarch slurry, cashew nuts, green onions, and sesame seeds in the Instant Pot.
2. Give a good stir.
3. Close the lid and press the Manual button.
4. Adjust the cooking time to 15 minutes.
5. Do quick pressure release.
6. Once the lid is open, press the Sauté button and stir in the slurry.
7. Allow simmering until the sauce thickens.
8. Stir in the cashew nuts, green onions, and sesame seeds last.

Nutrition information:
Calories per serving: 444; Carbohydrates: 10.5g; Protein: 27.6g; Fat: 32.1g; Fiber: 0.9g

40-Clove Chicken

Serves: 6
Preparation Time: 5 minutes
Cooking Time: 20 minutes
Ingredients
- 1 tablespoon olive oil
- 1 tablespoon butter
- 4 chicken thighs, bone and skin not removed
- 2 chicken breasts, bone and skin not removed
- Salt and pepper
- 40 cloves of garlic, peeled and sliced
- 2 sprigs of thyme
- ¼ cup dry white wine
- ¼ cup chicken broth
- Parsley for garnish

Instructions
1. Press the Sauté button on the Instant Pot.
2. Pour the oil and butter.
3. Stir in the chicken pieces and season with salt and pepper to taste.
4. Add the garlic cloves. Continue stirring for 5 minutes until fragrant.
5. Stir in the thyme, white wine, and chicken broth.
6. Place all ingredients except for the cornstarch slurry, sesame seeds, and green onions in the Instant Pot.
7. Give a good stir.
8. Close the lid and press the Manual button.
9. Adjust the cooking time to 15 minutes.
10. Do quick pressure release.
11. Once the lid is open, garnish with parsley.

Nutrition information:
Calories per serving: 549; Carbohydrates: 7.8g; Protein: 45.9g; Fat: 36.3g; Fiber: 0.2g

Instant Pot BBQ Chicken with Potatoes

Serves: 8
Preparation Time: 5 minutes
Cooking Time: 15 minutes
Ingredients
- 2 pounds chicken
- 1 cup BBQ sauce
- ½ cup water
- 1 tablespoon Italian seasoning
- 1 tablespoon minced garlic
- 3 large potatoes, peeled and chopped
- 1 large onion, sliced

Instructions
1. Place all ingredients in the Instant Pot.
2. Give a good stir.
3. Close the lid and press the Poultry button.
4. Adjust the cooking time to 15 minutes.
5. Do quick pressure release.

Nutrition information:
Calories per serving: 254; Carbohydrates: 29.1g; Protein: 26.7g; Fat: 3.3g; Fiber: 4.1g

Asian Garlic and Honey Chicken

Serves: 6
Preparation Time: 5 minutes
Cooking Time: 15 minutes
Ingredients
- 1 ½ pounds chicken breasts, cut into cubes
- 6 tablespoons honey
- 3 cloves of garlic, minced
- 2 tablespoons online powder
- 1 ½ tablespoons soy sauce
- ½ tablespoon sriracha sauce
- 1 cup water
- 1 tablespoon cornstarch + 2 tablespoons water
- Green onions, chopped
- 1 tablespoon sesame oil

Instructions
1. Place all ingredients except for the cornstarch slurry and green onions in the Instant Pot.
2. Give a good stir.
3. Close the lid and press the Poultry button.
4. Adjust the cooking time to 15 minutes.
5. Do quick pressure release.
6. Once the lid is open, press the Sauté button and stir in the cornstarch slurry.
7. Simmer until the sauce thickens.
8. Stir in green onions and sesame oil last.

Nutrition information:
Calories per serving: 296; Carbohydrates:19.6 g; Protein: 24.2g; Fat: 13.5g; Fiber: 0.4g

Mojo Chicken Tacos

Serves: 12
Preparation Time: 5 minutes
Cooking Time: 20 minutes
Ingredients
- ¼ cup olive oil
- 12 chicken breasts, skin and bones removed
- 8 cloves of garlic, minced
- 2/3 cup lime juice, freshly squeezed
- 2/3 cup orange juice, freshly squeezed
- 1 tablespoon orange peel
- 1 tablespoon dried oregano
- 2 tablespoons ground cumin
- Salt and pepper
- ¼ cup cilantro, chopped

Instructions
1. Press the Sauté button on the Instant Pot.
2. Stir in the chicken breasts and garlic. Cook until the chicken pieces have turned lightly brown.
3. Add the rest of the ingredients except for the cilantro.
4. Close the lid and press the Poultry button.
5. Adjust the cooking time to 15 minutes.
6. Do quick pressure release.
7. Garnish with cilantro.

Nutrition information:
Calories per serving: 558; Carbohydrates: 4.5g; Protein: 60.8g; Fat: 31.6g; Fiber: 0.4g

Instant Pot Orange Chicken

Serves: 4
Preparation Time: 5 minutes
Cooking Time: 15 minutes
Ingredients
- 4 chicken breasts
- ¾ cup barbecue sauce
- 2 tablespoons soy sauce
- ¾ cup orange marmalade
- ¼ cup water
- 1 tablespoon cornstarch + 2 tablespoons water
- 2 tablespoons green onions, chopped

Instructions
1. Place all ingredients except for the cornstarch slurry and green onions in the Instant Pot.
2. Give a good stir.
3. Close the lid and press the Poultry button.
4. Adjust the cooking time to 15 minutes.
5. Do quick pressure release.
6. Once the lid is open, press the Sauté button and stir in the cornstarch slurry.
7. Simmer until the sauce thickens.
8. Stir in green onions last.

Nutrition information:
Calories per serving:763; Carbohydrates: 63.8g; Protein: 61.7g; Fat: 28.6g; Fiber: 1.1g

Belizean Stewed Chicken

Serves: 8
Preparation Time: 5 minutes
Cooking Time: 15 minutes
Ingredients
- 1 tablespoon coconut oil
- 1 onion, sliced
- 3 cloves of garlic, minced
- 4 whole chicken legs
- 2 tablespoons achiote seasoning
- 2 tablespoons white vinegar
- 3 tablespoons Worcestershire sauce
- 1 teaspoon ground cumin

- 1 teaspoon dried oregano
- Salt and pepper to taste
- 1 tablespoon granulated sugar
- 2 cups chicken stock

Instructions
1. Press the Sauté button and pour oil into the Instant Pot.
2. Sauté the onion, garlic, and chicken. Continue stirring until all sides turn golden brown.
3. Stir in the rest of the ingredients.
4. Close the lid and press the Poultry button.
5. Adjust the cooking time to 15 minutes.
6. Do quick pressure release.

Nutrition information:
Calories per serving: 279; Carbohydrates:1.8g; Protein: 28g; Fat: 18g; Fiber: 0g

Lazy Sweet and Sour Chicken

Serves: 8
Preparation Time: 5 minutes
Cooking Time: 15 minutes

Ingredients
- 2 pounds chicken meat
- 4 cloves of garlic, minced
- 1 onion, chopped
- 1 green bell pepper, julienned
- ½ cup ketchup
- ½ cup molasses
- ¼ cup soy sauce
- 1 tablespoon cornstarch + 2 tablespoons water

Instructions
1. Press the Sauté button on the Instant Pot.
2. Place the chicken, garlic, and onion. Stir to combine everything and until the chicken meat has turned lightly golden.
3. Stir in the bell pepper, ketchup, molasses, and soy sauce.
4. Close the lid and press the Poultry button.
5. Adjust the cooking time to 15 minutes.
6. Do quick pressure release.
7. Once the lid is open, press the Sauté button and stir in the cornstarch slurry.
8. Allow simmering until the sauce thickens.

Nutrition information:
Calories per serving: 287; Carbohydrates: 24.1g; Protein: 23.4g; Fat: 10.7g; Fiber: 0.6g

Chicken with White Wine Mushroom Sauce

Serves: 12
Preparation Time: 5 minutes
Cooking Time: 20 minutes

Ingredients
- 2 tablespoons vegetable oil
- 6 chicken breasts, halved
- 1 onion, chopped
- 4 cloves of garlic, minced
- 1 ¼ pounds cremini mushrooms, sliced
- 1 ½ cups dry white wine
- 1 cup chicken broth
- 1 tablespoon thyme
- 2 bay leaves
- 1 tablespoon lemon juice, freshly squeezed
- Salt and pepper
- 2 tablespoons cornstarch + 2 tablespoons water

Instructions
1. Press the Sauté button on the Instant Pot.
2. Heat the oil and place the chicken.
3. Add the onion and garlic. Stir to combine everything and until the chicken meat has turned lightly golden.
4. Stir in the mushrooms, dry white wine, broth, thyme, bay leaves, and lemon juice. Season with salt and pepper to taste.
5. Close the lid and press the Poultry button.
6. Adjust the cooking time to 15 minutes.
7. Do quick pressure release.
8. Once the lid is open, press the Sauté button and stir in the cornstarch slurry.
9. Allow simmering until the sauce thickens.

Nutrition information:
Calories per serving: 487; Carbohydrates: 37.7g; Protein: 42.3g; Fat: 20.5g; Fiber: 5.7g

Instant Pot Jamaican Jerk Chicken

Serves: 6
Preparation Time: 5 minutes
Cooking Time: 15 minutes

Ingredients
- 6 chicken drumsticks
- ½ cup ketchup
- ¼ cup dark brown sugar
- ¼ cup red wine vinegar
- 3 tablespoons soy sauce
- 2 tablespoons Jamaican jerk seasoning
- Salt and pepper to taste

Instructions
1. Place all ingredients in the Instant Pot.
2. Give a good stir to coat the chicken.
3. Close the lid and press the Poultry button.
4. Adjust the cooking time to 15 minutes.
5. Do quick pressure release.

Nutrition information:
Calories per serving: 209; Carbohydrates: 9g; Protein: 11g; Fat: 3g; Fiber: 7g

Instant Pot Chicken Creole

Serves: 6
Preparation Time: 5 minutes
Cooking Time: 15 minutes

Ingredients
- ½ cup butter
- 4 chicken breasts, boneless
- 1 cup chopped onion
- ½ cup chopped celery
- ½ cup green bell pepper, chopped
- 1 teaspoon coconut sugar
- ¼ teaspoon ground cloves
- 1 teaspoon garlic powder
- ½ teaspoon white pepper

- ½ teaspoon black pepper
- ½ teaspoon cayenne pepper
- ½ teaspoon dried basil
- 1 cup chopped tomatoes
- 1 cup tomato sauce
- 1 cup chicken broth
- Salt to taste

Instructions
1. Press the Sauté button on the Instant Pot.
2. Heat the butter and stir in the chicken breasts, onion, and celery. Stir until fragrant and the chicken lightly brown.
3. Add the rest of the ingredients.
4. Scrape the bottom of the pot to remove the browning.
5. Close the lid and press the Poultry button.
6. Adjust the cooking time to 15 minutes.
7. Do quick pressure release.

Nutrition information:
Calories per serving:599; Carbohydrates: 13.9g; Protein: 50.8g; Fat: 36.3g; Fiber: 3.7g

Instant Pot Chicken Piccata

Serves: 6
Preparation Time: 5 minutes
Cooking Time: 15 minutes

Ingredients
- 1 ½ pounds chicken breasts, bones, and skin removed
- 2 teaspoons salt
- ½ cup all-purpose flour
- 2 tablespoons olive oil
- 3 cloves of garlic, minced
- ¾ cup chicken broth
- 1/3 cup lemon juice, freshly squeezed
- 1 sprig of basil, chopped
- 3 ounces capers, drained
- ¼ cup sour cream

Instructions
1. Season the chicken breasts with 1 teaspoon of salt.
2. Place in a Ziploc bag and pour in flour. Dredge the chicken pieces in the flour. Set aside.
3. Press the Sauté button on the Instant Pot.
4. Add the olive oil and place the dredged chicken pieces inside. Sear on both sides until lightly brown.
5. Add the garlic and allow to sauté for 30 seconds.
6. Stir in the chicken broth, lemon juice, basil, and capers.
7. Season with the remaining salt.
8. Close the lid and press the Poultry button.
9. Adjust the cooking time to 10 minutes.
10. Do quick pressure release.
11. Serve with sour cream.

Nutrition information:
Calories per serving:342; Carbohydrates: 10.2g; Protein: 32.1g; Fat: 18.4g; Fiber: 0.8g

Root Beer Chicken Wings

Serves: 8
Preparation Time: 5 minutes
Cooking Time: 15 minutes

Ingredients
- 2 pounds chicken wings
- 2 cans of root beer
- ¼ cup sugar
- ¼ cup soy sauce

Instructions
1. Place all ingredients in the Instant Pot.
2. Give a good stir.
3. Close the lid and press the Poultry button.
4. Adjust the cooking time to 10 minutes.
5. Do quick pressure release.

Nutrition information:
Calories per serving: 229; Carbohydrates: 18.2g; Protein:25.5 g; Fat: 5.5g; Fiber: 0.2g

Instant Pot Alfredo Chicken Noodles

Serves: 4
Preparation Time: 5 minutes
Cooking Time: 15 minutes

Ingredients
- 1 tablespoon olive oil
- 2 chicken breasts, bones, and skin removed
- Salt and pepper
- 5 cloves of garlic, minced
- 2 tablespoons butter
- 2 cups heavy cream
- 2 cups chicken broth
- A pinch of ground nutmeg
- 1 package dry fettuccini noodles
- ½ cup parmesan cheese, grated
- Fresh basil leaves for garnish

Instructions
1. Press the Sauté button on the Instant Pot.
2. Pour the oil and sauté the chicken breasts. Season with salt and pepper. Cook until lightly brown.
3. Stir in the garlic until fragrant.
4. Add the butter, heavy cream, broth, nutmeg, and noodles.
5. Close the lid and press the Poultry button.
6. Adjust the cooking time to 10 minutes.
7. Do quick pressure release.
8. Do natural pressure release.
9. Open the lid and garnish with parmesan cheese and basil.

Nutrition information:
Calories per serving: 571; Carbohydrates: 10.5g; Protein: 38.6g; Fat: 50.3g; Fiber: 0.9g

Chicken with Mushrooms and Mustard

Serves: 4
Preparation Time: 5 minutes
Cooking Time: 15 minutes

Ingredients
- 4 chicken breasts, halved
- 2 tablespoons flour
- 2 tablespoon vegetable oil
- 1 tablespoon butter
- 1 onion, chopped
- 1 cup mushrooms, sliced

- ½ cup light cream
- 1 tablespoon fresh parsley, chopped
- 1 tablespoon Dijon mustard
- 1 tablespoon lemon juice, freshly squeezed
- Salt and pepper

Instructions
1. Pound the chicken breasts and dredge in the flour. Set aside.
2. Press the Sauté button on the Instant Pot.
3. Heat the oil and butter and add the dredged chicken pieces. Cook on all sides for 3 minutes each.
4. Add the rest of the ingredients.
5. Close the lid and press the Poultry button.
6. Adjust the cooking time to 10 minutes.
7. Do quick pressure release.

Nutrition information:
Calories per serving: 675; Carbohydrates: 8.4g; Protein: 62.4g; Fat: 42.6g; Fiber:1 g

Quick Hoisin Chicken

Serves: 6
Preparation Time: 5 minutes
Cooking Time: 15 minutes

Ingredients
- 6 ounces snow peas
- 1 can water chestnuts, cut into quarters
- 1-pound chicken breasts, cut into bite-sized pieces
- Salt and pepper to taste
- 4 tablespoons hoisin sauce
- 2 teaspoons sugar
- ¼ cup soy sauce
- 1 tablespoon cornstarch + 2 tablespoons water

Instructions
1. Place all ingredients in the Instant Pot except for the cornstarch slurry.
2. Close the lid and press the Poultry button.
3. Adjust the cooking time to 15 minutes.
4. Do quick pressure release.
5. Once the lid is open, press the Sauté button and stir in the cornstarch slurry.
6. Simmer until the sauce thickens.

Nutrition information:
Calories per serving: 240; Carbohydrates:19.2 g; Protein: 18.5g; Fat:9.5g; Fiber:1.4g

Sticky Chicken and Chilies

Serves: 8
Preparation Time: 5 minutes
Cooking Time: 15 minutes

Ingredients
- 8 chicken thighs
- ¼ cup honey
- 1 ½ tablespoons chili paste
- ½ cup chicken broth
- 2 cloves of garlic, minced
- 2 tablespoons currants
- 2 tablespoon olive oil
- 2 tablespoons balsamic vinegar
- Rind from 1 small lemon

Instructions
1. Place all ingredients in the Instant Pot except for the cornstarch slurry.
2. Close the lid and press the Poultry button.
3. Adjust the cooking time to 15 minutes.
4. Do quick pressure release.

Nutrition information:
Calories per serving:522; Carbohydrates: 11.5g; Protein: 35.5g; Fat: 36.9g; Fiber: 0.6g

Instant Pot Herbed Chicken

Serves: 4
Preparation Time: 5 minutes
Cooking Time: 15 minutes

Ingredients
- 4 chicken breasts, halved
- 1 package herb sprinkle of your choice
- 1 ½ cups long-grain rice
- 3 cups chicken broth
- 2 tablespoons oregano leaves
- Salt and pepper

Instructions
1. Season the chicken breasts with the herbs of your choice. Set aside.
2. Pour the rice, chicken broth, and oregano in the Instant Pot.
3. Season with salt and pepper.
4. Place the chicken meat on top.
5. Close the lid and press the Poultry button.
6. Adjust the cooking time to 15 minutes.
7. Do quick pressure release.

Nutrition information:
Calories per serving: 774; Carbohydrates: 55.7g; Protein: 69.3g; Fat: 28.9g; Fiber:2.9g

Yakitori Chicken Wings

Serves: 12
Preparation Time: 5 minutes
Cooking Time: 15 minutes

Ingredients
- ½ cup yakitori sauce
- 2 cloves of garlic, minced
- 1 thumb-size ginger, grated
- 12 chicken wings
- ½ cup water
- 1 green onion, chopped
- ½ teaspoon sesame seeds, toasted

Instructions
1. Place the yakitori sauce, garlic, ginger, and chicken wings in the Instant Pot.
2. Pour in water and give a good stir.
3. Close the lid and press the Poultry button.
4. Adjust the cooking time to 15 minutes.
5. Do quick pressure release.
6. Once the lid is open, garnish with green onions and sesame seeds.

Nutrition information:
Calories per serving: 266; Carbohydrates: 2.9g; Protein: 15.7g; Fat: 5.9g; Fiber:0.2g

Balsamic Orange Chicken Drumsticks

Serves: 8
Preparation Time: 5 minutes
Cooking Time: 20 minutes
Ingredients
- 1 tablespoon olive oil
- 8 chicken drumsticks
- 2 tablespoons balsamic vinegar
- 1/3 cup orange marmalade
- 1/3 cup orange juice, freshly squeezed
- 2 tablespoons honey

Instructions
1. Press the Sauté button on the Instant Pot.
2. Heat the oil and place the chicken drumsticks. Stir to brown all edges.
3. Pour in the rest of the ingredients.
4. Close the lid and press the Poultry button.
5. Adjust the cooking time to 15 minutes.
6. Do quick pressure release.

Nutrition information:
Calories per serving: 281; Carbohydrates: 15.1g; Protein: 26.3g; Fat: 13.7g; Fiber: 0.1g

French Style Chicken Potatoes

Serves: 8
Preparation Time: 5 minutes
Cooking Time: 20 minutes
Ingredients
- 1 tablespoon unsalted butter
- 4 chicken thighs
- 2 cloves of garlic, minced
- 1 onion, chopped
- 1 teaspoon onion powder
- 1 teaspoon garlic powder
- 2 teaspoons white sugar
- ¼ cup Dijon mustard
- 1 teaspoon rosemary
- 1 teaspoon thyme
- ½ pound baby potatoes, scrubbed and halved
- Salt and pepper
- 1 cup dry white wine
- ½ cup chicken stock
- 2 tablespoons flour + 2 tablespoons milk

Instructions
1. Press the Sauté button on the Instant Pot.
2. Melt the butter and add the chicken thighs, garlic, and onion. Stir to brown the chicken meat and until fragrant.
3. Add the onion powder, garlic powder, sugar, mustard, rosemary, thyme, and baby potatoes. Season with salt and pepper to taste. Continue stirring for 2 minutes.
4. Pour into the dry white wine and chicken stock.
5. Close the lid and press the Poultry button.
6. Adjust the cooking time to 15 minutes.
7. Do quick pressure release.
8. Once the lid is open, press the Sauté button.
9. Stir in the flour mixture and allow to simmer until the sauce thickens.

Nutrition information:
Calories per serving: 308; Carbohydrates:9.4g; Protein: 20.8g; Fat: 20.7g; Fiber: 1.4g

Stocks and Sauces Recipes

Basic Vegetable Stock

Serves: 12
Preparation Time: 3 minutes
Cooking Time: 15 minutes
Ingredients
- 1 onion, chopped
- 2 stalks of celery, roughly chopped
- 2 carrots, cut into chunks
- 8 cloves of garlic, crushed
- 8 sprigs fresh thyme
- 8 sprigs parsley
- 2 bay leaves
- 1 teaspoon salt
- 6 cups water

Instructions
1. Place all ingredients in the Instant Pot.
2. Close the lid and press the Manual button.
3. Adjust the cooking time to 15 minutes
4. Do natural pressure release.
5. Run the stock through a sieve and discard the vegetables.
6. Place in mason jars and store in the fridge until ready to serve.

Nutrition information:
Calories per serving: 12; Carbohydrates: 2.6g; Protein: 0.4g; Fat: 0g; Fiber: 0.5g

Turkey Giblet Stock

Serves: 12
Preparation Time: 5 minutes
Cooking Time: 45 minutes
Ingredients
- 1 bag turkey giblet
- 6 cups water
- 1 stalk of celery, sliced
- 1 carrot, sliced
- 1 onion, quartered
- 1 bay leaf
- 1 teaspoon whole black peppercorns

Instructions
1. Place all ingredients in the Instant Pot.
2. Close the lid and press the Manual button.
3. Adjust the cooking time to 45 minutes
4. Do natural pressure release.
5. Run the stock through a sieve and discard the solids.
6. Place in mason jars and store in the fridge until ready to serve.

Nutrition information:
Calories per serving: 20; Carbohydrates: 0.9g; Protein: 2.5g; Fat: 0.7g; Fiber: 0.2g

Basic Beef Stock

Serves: 12
Preparation Time: 5 minutes
Cooking Time: 60 minutes
Ingredients
- 6 pounds beef soup bones
- 1 onion, chopped
- 3 carrots, chopped
- 12 cups water
- 2 stalks celery, sliced
- 1 tomato, chopped
- 8 whole peppercorns
- 1 bay leaf
- 1 teaspoon salt

Instructions
1. Place all ingredients in the Instant Pot.
2. Close the lid and press the Manual button.
3. Adjust the cooking time to 60 minutes
4. Do natural pressure release.
5. Run the stock through a sieve and discard the solids.
6. Place in mason jars and store in the fridge until ready to serve.

Nutrition information:
Calories per serving: 238; Carbohydrates: 2.8g; Protein: 22.9g; Fat: 14.3g; Fiber: 0.8g

Asian Chicken Stock

Serves: 14
Preparation Time: 3 minutes
Cooking Time: 45 minutes
Ingredients
- 4 pounds chicken
- 7 cups water
- 1 onion, halved
- 3 stalks of celery, sliced
- 3 carrots, chopped
- 1 bay leaf
- 1 thumb-sized ginger, sliced

Instructions
1. Place all ingredients in the Instant Pot.
2. Close the lid and press the Manual button.
3. Adjust the cooking time to 45 minutes
4. Do natural pressure release.
5. Run the stock through a sieve and discard the solids.
6. Place in mason jars and store in the fridge until ready to serve.

Nutrition information:
Calories per serving: 153; Carbohydrates: 2.1g; Protein: 26.5g; Fat: 3.5g; Fiber: 0.6g

Simple Bone Broth

Serves: 8
Preparation Time: 3 minutes
Cooking Time: 60 minutes
Ingredients
- 2 pounds beef bones
- 6 cups water
- 2 onions, sliced
- 3 cloves of garlic, crushed
- 2 carrots, chopped
- 1 bay leaf

Instructions
1. Place all ingredients in the Instant Pot.
2. Close the lid and press the Manual button.
3. Adjust the cooking time to 60 minutes
4. Do natural pressure release.
5. Run the stock through a sieve and discard the solids.

6. Place in mason jars and store in the fridge until ready to serve.
Nutrition information:
Calories per serving: 249; Carbohydrates: 2.1g; Protein: 31.9g; Fat: 11.8g; Fiber: 0.5g

Japanese Dashi Stock

Serves: 12
Preparation Time: 2 minutes
Cooking Time: 60 minutes
Ingredients
- 1-ounce dashi kombu or dried kelp
- 6 cups water
- ½ cup bonito flakes

Instructions
1. Place all ingredients in the Instant Pot.
2. Close the lid and press the Manual button.
3. Adjust the cooking time to 60 minutes
4. Do natural pressure release.
5. Run the stock through a sieve and discard the solids.
6. Place in mason jars and store in the fridge until ready to serve.
Nutrition information:
Calories per serving: 22; Carbohydrates: 3.4g; Protein: 0.3g; Fat: 1g; Fiber: 0.6g

Instant Pot Scotch Broth

Serves: 8
Preparation Time: 3 minutes
Cooking Time: 60 minutes
Ingredients
- 2 ¼ pounds leg of lamb
- 8 cups water
- 3 onions, chopped
- 3 turnips, chopped
- 1 carrot, chopped
- 1 teaspoon whole black peppercorns
- ½ cup barley
- 1 bay leaf

Instructions
1. Place all ingredients in the Instant Pot.
2. Close the lid and press the Manual button.
3. Adjust the cooking time to 60 minutes
4. Do natural pressure release.
5. Run the stock through a sieve and discard the solids.
6. Place in mason jars and store in the fridge until ready to serve.
Nutrition information:
Calories per serving: 235; Carbohydrates: 14.3g; Protein: 27.7g; Fat: 6.9g; Fiber: 2.9g

Smoked Turkey Stock

Serves: 12
Preparation Time: 3 minutes
Cooking Time: 60 minutes
Ingredients
- 2 smoked turkey legs
- 1 onion, cut in half
- 1 carrot, chopped
- 1 large bell pepper, chopped
- 9 cups of water
- 5 cloves of garlic, crushed
- 10 whole black peppercorns
- Salt and pepper

Instructions
1. Place all ingredients in the Instant Pot.
2. Close the lid and press the Manual button.
3. Adjust the cooking time to 60 minutes
4. Do natural pressure release.
5. Run the stock through a sieve and discard the solids.
6. Place in mason jars and store in the fridge until ready to serve.
Nutrition information:
Calories per serving: 200; Carbohydrates: 2.5g; Protein: 25.7g; Fat: 8.9g; Fiber: 0.2g

Instant Pot White Stock

Serves: 8
Preparation Time: 2 minutes
Cooking Time: 60 minutes
Ingredients
- 3 pounds chicken
- 1 veal knuckle
- 2 stalks of celery, sliced
- 1 onion, chopped
- 8 cups water
- Salt and pepper

Instructions
1. Place all ingredients in the Instant Pot.
2. Close the lid and press the Manual button.
3. Adjust the cooking time to 60 minutes
4. Do natural pressure release.
5. Run the stock through a sieve and discard the solids.
6. Place in mason jars and store in the fridge until ready to serve.
Nutrition information:
Calories per serving: 216; Carbohydrates: 1.9g; Protein: 38.1g; Fat: 5.1g; Fiber: 0.4g

Hoshi Shiitake Dashi

Serves: 4
Preparation Time: 3 minutes
Cooking Time: 25 minutes
Ingredients
- 4 cups water
- 4 dried shiitake mushrooms, soaked in water then rinsed

Instructions
1. Place all ingredients in the Instant Pot.
2. Close the lid and press the Manual button.
3. Adjust the cooking time to 25 minutes
4. Do natural pressure release.
5. Run the stock through a sieve and discard the solids.
6. Place in mason jars and store in the fridge until ready to serve.
Nutrition information:
Calories per serving: 10; Carbohydrates: 2.5g; Protein: 0.3g; Fat: 0g; Fiber: 0.4g

Vegan and Gluten-Free Stock

Serves: 8

Preparation Time: 3 minutes
Cooking Time: 30 minutes
Ingredients
- 4 stalks celery, sliced
- 2 carrots, chopped
- 1 onion, quartered
- 2 shallots, halved
- 1 fennel bulb, sliced thickly
- 1/8 apple, cored and sliced
- 10 whole black peppercorns
- 1 bay leaf
- 8 cups water

Instructions
1. Place all ingredients in the Instant Pot.
2. Close the lid and press the Manual button.
3. Adjust the cooking time to 30 minutes
4. Do natural pressure release.
5. Run the stock through a sieve and discard the solids.
6. Place in mason jars and store in the fridge until ready to serve.

Nutrition information:
Calories per serving:24; Carbohydrates: 5.5g; Protein:0.7 g; Fat: 0.1g; Fiber: 1.8g

Mushroom Gravy Sauce

Serves: 8
Preparation Time: 3 minutes
Cooking Time: 8 minutes
Ingredients
- 2 tablespoons butter
- 1 package button mushrooms, sliced
- ¼ cup shallots, chopped
- 2 tablespoons flour
- 2 cups beef broth
- ¼ cup half and half
- ½ teaspoon ground black pepper
- Salt

Instructions
1. Press the Sauté button and melt the butter.
2. Sauté the mushrooms and shallots until fragrant.
3. Using a whisk, stir in the flour and broth. Whisk until smooth.
4. Allow simmering for 5 minutes.
5. Stir in the half and half. Season with pepper and salt.
6. Close the lid and press the Manual button.
7. Adjust the cooking time to 3 minutes.
8. Do natural pressure release.

Nutrition information:
Calories per serving: 63; Carbohydrates: 8.3g; Protein: 0.9g; Fat:3.1 g; Fiber: 0.3g

Asian Soup Stock

Serves: 10
Preparation Time: 3 minutes
Cooking Time: 25 minutes
Ingredients
- 10 cups water
- 2 onions, chopped
- 5 carrots, sliced
- 3 stalks celery, sliced
- 10 cloves garlic
- 6 whole cloves
- 1 ginger, sliced
- 5 dried shiitake mushrooms, soaked
- ½ teaspoon salt

Instructions
1. Place all ingredients in the Instant Pot.
2. Close the lid and press the Manual button.
3. Adjust the cooking time to 25 minutes
4. Do natural pressure release.
5. Run the stock through a sieve and discard the solids.
6. Place in mason jars and store in the fridge until ready to serve.

Nutrition information:
Calories per serving: 20; Carbohydrates: 4.6g; Protein: 0.6g; Fat: 0g; Fiber: 0.8g

Turkey Soup Stock

Serves: 8
Preparation Time: 3 minutes
Cooking Time: 45 minutes
Ingredients
- 1-pound turkey bones
- 4 cups carrots, cut into chunks
- 3 cups onion, quartered
- 3 cups parsnips, chopped
- 5 cups celery, sliced
- 2 teaspoons dried sage
- 2 teaspoons dried thyme
- 4 bay leaves
- 1 teaspoon whole peppercorns
- 8 cups water

Instructions
1. Place all ingredients in the Instant Pot.
2. Close the lid and press the Manual button.
3. Adjust the cooking time to 45 minutes
4. Do natural pressure release.
5. Run the stock through a sieve and discard the solids.
6. Place in mason jars and store in the fridge until ready to serve.

Nutrition information:
Calories per serving:185; Carbohydrates: 20.3g; Protein: 18.8g; Fat:3.3 g; Fiber: 5.8g

Thai Soup Stock

Serves: 8
Preparation Time: 3 minutes
Cooking Time: 45 minutes
Ingredients
- 8 cups water
- 1-pound chicken bones
- 1 onion, quartered
- 1 cup fresh cilantro, chopped
- 2 stalks lemongrass
- 2 kaffir lime leaves
- 1 tablespoon sliced ginger
- ½ teaspoon salt

- ½ teaspoon whole peppercorns

Instructions
1. Place all ingredients in the Instant Pot.
2. Close the lid and press the Manual button.
3. Adjust the cooking time to 45 minutes
4. Do natural pressure release.
5. Run the stock through a sieve and discard the solids.
6. Place in mason jars and store in the fridge until ready to serve.

Nutrition information:
Calories per serving: 72; Carbohydrates: 2.4g; Protein: 11.8g; Fat:1.6 g; Fiber: 0.3g

Chinese Pork Stock

Serves: 8
Preparation Time: 3 minutes
Cooking time: 60 minutes
Ingredients
- 2 pounds pork leg bones
- 2 tablespoons Shaoxing wine
- 1 thumb-size ginger, crushed
- 2 star anise
- 1 bay leaf
- 8 cups water

Instructions
1. Place all ingredients in the Instant Pot.
2. Close the lid and press the Manual button.
3. Adjust the cooking time to 60 minutes
4. Do natural pressure release.
5. Run the stock through a sieve and discard the solids.
6. Place in mason jars and store in the fridge until ready to serve.

Nutrition information:
Calories per serving: 61; Carbohydrates: 0.3g; Protein: 11.1g; Fat: 0.6g; Fiber: 0g

Classic Pork Broth

Serves: 8
Preparation Time: 3 minutes
Cooking Time: 60 minutes
Ingredients
- 3 pounds pork bones
- 1 tablespoon apple cider vinegar
- 1 teaspoon whole peppercorns
- Salt to taste

Instructions
1. Place all ingredients in the Instant Pot.
2. Close the lid and press the Manual button.
3. Adjust the cooking time to 60 minutes
4. Do natural pressure release.
5. Run the stock through a sieve and discard the solids.
6. Place in mason jars and store in the fridge until ready to serve.

Nutrition information:
Calories per serving:357; Carbohydrates: 0.3g; Protein: 43.5g; Fat: 18.8g; Fiber: 0g

Seafood Soup Stock

Serves: 8
Preparation Time: 3 minutes
Cooking Time: 30 minutes
Ingredients
- 8 cups water
- 4 carrots, sliced
- Shells and heads from ½ pound prawns
- 4 onions, quartered
- 2 bay leaves
- 3 cloves of garlic
- 5 whole cloves
- 1 teaspoon black pepper

Instructions
1. Place all ingredients in the Instant Pot.
2. Close the lid and press the Manual button.
3. Adjust the cooking time to 30 minutes
4. Do natural pressure release.
5. Run the stock through a sieve and discard the solids.
6. Place in mason jars and store in the fridge until ready to serve.

Nutrition information:
Calories per serving: 128; Carbohydrates: 12.3g; Protein: 3.2g; Fat: 7.4g; Fiber: 1.3g

Easy Venison Broth

Serves: 8
Preparation Time: 3 minutes
Cooking Time: 1 hour and 30 minutes
Ingredients
- 4 pounds venison bones
- Salt
- 1 tablespoon juniper berries
- 2 tablespoons rosemary
- 1 tablespoon black peppercorns
- Bay leaves
- 1 onion, chopped
- 2 stalks of celery, sliced
- 1 carrot, chopped

Instructions
1. Place all ingredients in the Instant Pot.
2. Close the lid and press the Manual button.
3. Adjust the cooking time to 1 hour and 30 minutes
4. Do natural pressure release.
5. Run the stock through a sieve and discard the solids.
6. Place in mason jars and store in the fridge until ready to serve.

Nutrition information:
Calories per serving: 140; Carbohydrates: 2.4g; Protein: 11.6g; Fat: 9.2g; Fiber: 0.6g

Instant Pot Herb Stock

Serves: 4
Preparation Time: 3 minutes
Cooking Time: 15 minutes
Ingredients
- A handful of rosemary,
- 1 sprig of parsley

- 3 bay leaves
- 2 cloves of garlic, crushed
- 1 teaspoon black peppercorns
- 4 cups water

Instructions
1. Place all ingredients in the Instant Pot.
2. Close the lid and press the Manual button.
3. Adjust the cooking time to 15 minutes
4. Do natural pressure release.
5. Run the stock through a sieve and discard the solids.
6. Place in mason jars and store in the fridge until ready to serve.

Nutrition information:
Calories per serving:3; Carbohydrates: 0.6g; Protein: 0.1g; Fat: 0g; Fiber: 0g

Korean-Style Dashi Stock

Serves: 6
Preparation Time: 3 minutes
Cooking Time: 25 minutes

Ingredients
- 6 cups water
- 10 grams dried kelp or Japanese Kombu
- ¼ cup dried anchovies, guts removed

Instructions
1. Place all ingredients in the Instant Pot.
2. Close the lid and press the Manual button.
3. Adjust the cooking time to 25 minutes
4. Do natural pressure release.
5. Run the stock through a sieve and discard the solids.
6. Place in mason jars and store in the fridge until ready to serve.

Nutrition information:
Calories per serving: 4; Carbohydrates: 1.1g; Protein: 0.9g; Fat: 0g; Fiber: 0.1g

Vietnamese Pho Stock

Serves: 4
Preparation Time: 3 minutes
Cooking Time: 45 minutes

Ingredients
- 2 onions, chopped
- 4-inch piece ginger, sliced
- 2 whole cinnamon sticks
- 2 whole star anise
- 3 whole cloves
- 2 teaspoons whole coriander seeds
- 6 cups beef broth
- 1 tablespoon soy sauce
- 1 tablespoon fish sauce
- 3 carrots, peeled and chopped

Instructions
1. On a stove top, char the onions and ginger for five minutes on each side. Rinse the onions and ginger under cool running water.
2. Press the Sauté button on the Instant Pot.
3. Place the cinnamon sticks, star anise, cloves, and coriander seeds and dry roast for 2 minutes until they become toasty and fragrant.
4. Pour in the rest of the ingredients including the charred onions and ginger.
5. Close the lid and press the Manual button.
6. Adjust the cooking time to 45 minutes
7. Do natural pressure release.
8. Run the stock through a sieve and discard the solids.
9. Place in mason jars and store in the fridge until ready to serve.

Nutrition information:
Calories per serving:197; Carbohydrates: 43.2g; Protein: 4.1g; Fat: 1.6g; Fiber: 3.2g

Roasted Chicken Stock

Serves: 8
Preparation Time: 3 minutes
Cooking Time: 30 minutes

Ingredients
- 1-pound chicken bones
- 10 cups water
- 2 onions, peeled
- 1 leek, washed and sliced
- 4 stalks of celery, minced
- 2 carrots, chopped
- 2 bay leaves
- 8 cloves of garlic, crushed
- ½ teaspoon whole peppercorns
- 2 sprigs thyme

Instructions
1. Place all ingredients in the Instant Pot.
2. Close the lid and press the Manual button.
3. Adjust the cooking time to 30 minutes
4. Do natural pressure release.
5. Run the stock through a sieve and discard the solids.
6. Place in mason jars and store in the fridge until ready to serve.

Nutrition information:
Calories per serving:93; Carbohydrates: 6.8g; Protein: 12.4g; Fat: 1.7g; Fiber: 1.3g

Magic Mineral Broth

Serves: 6
Preparation Time: 3 minutes
Cooking Time: 40 minutes

Ingredients
- 6 carrots, unpeeled and sliced
- 2 onions, unpeeled and halved
- 1 leek, cut into thirds
- 1 bunch celery, cut into thirds
- 2 unpeeled Japanese sweet potatoes, quartered
- 5 cloves of garlic, crushed
- 1 strip of dried kelp or kombu
- 12 black peppercorns
- 2 bay leaves
- 8 cups water
- 1 teaspoon salt

Instructions
1. Place all ingredients in the Instant Pot.
2. Close the lid and press the Manual button.
3. Adjust the cooking time to 40 minutes
4. Do natural pressure release.
5. Run the stock through a sieve and discard the solids.
6. Place in mason jars and store in the fridge until ready to serve.
Nutrition information:
Calories per serving:45; Carbohydrates: 11g; Protein: 1g; Fat: 0.5g; Fiber: 2g

Instant Pot Shellfish Stock

Serves: 6
Preparation Time: 5 minutes
Cooking Time: 25 minutes
Ingredients
- 2 tablespoons olive oil
- 1 ¾ cups shallots, chopped
- 2 bulbs garlic, crushed
- 2 cups fennel bulb, sliced
- 1 cup sliced carrots
- 1 cup dry white wine
- A sprig of thyme
- 8 tarragon sprigs
- 6 parsley sprigs
- ½ teaspoon black peppercorns
- 1 tablespoon saffron threads
- 1-pound mussels
- 1-pound clams
- 1-pound oysters
- 10 cups water

Instructions
1. Press the Sauté button on the Instant Pot and heat the oil.
2. Sauté the shallots, garlic, and fennel bulbs until fragrant.
3. Add the rest of the ingredients.
4. Close the lid and press the Manual button.
5. Adjust the cooking time to 25 minutes
6. Do natural pressure release.
7. Run the stock through a sieve and discard the solids.
8. Place in mason jars and store in the fridge until ready to serve.
Nutrition information:
Calories per serving:286; Carbohydrates: 23.8g; Protein: 20.3g; Fat: 12.3g; Fiber: 3.4g

Instant Pot Cranberry Sauce

Serves: 6
Preparation Time: 3 minutes
Cooking Time: 5 minutes
Ingredients
- 1 bag cranberries
- Zest and juice of 1 lemon
- Zest and juice from 1 orange
- 1 apple, cored and chopped
- 10 strawberries, hulled and chopped
- ½ cup sugar
- 1 cinnamon stick

Instructions
1. Place all ingredients in the Instant Pot.
2. Close the lid and press the Manual button.
3. Adjust the cooking time to 5 minutes
4. Do natural pressure release.
Nutrition information:
Calories per serving: 91; Carbohydrates: 23.8g; Protein: 0.5g; Fat: 0.2g; Fiber: 4.6g

Instant Pot Strawberry Applesauce

Serves: 6
Preparation Time: 3 minutes
Cooking Time: 5 minutes
Ingredients
- 8 peeled apples, cored and sliced
- 3 cups strawberries, hulled and chopped
- ¼ teaspoon cinnamon powder
- 2 tablespoons lemon juice

Instructions
1. Place all ingredients in the Instant Pot.
2. Close the lid and press the Manual button.
3. Adjust the cooking time to 5 minutes
4. Do natural pressure release.
5. Place in mason jars.
Nutrition information:
Calories per serving: 151; Carbohydrates: 39.4g; Protein:1.1 g; Fat: 0.6g; Fiber: 7.3g

Instant Pot Mushroom Broth

Serves: 6
Preparation Time: 3 minutes
Cooking Time: 15 minutes
Ingredients
- 3 ounces dried mushrooms, soaked and rinsed
- 1 onion, quartered
- ½ cup carrots, chopped
- ½ cup celery, chopped
- 4 cloves of garlic, crushed
- 4 bay leaves
- 8 cups water

Instructions
1. Place all ingredients in the Instant Pot.
2. Close the lid and press the Manual button.
3. Adjust the cooking time to 15 minutes
4. Do natural pressure release.
5. Run the stock through a sieve and discard the solids.
6. Place in mason jars and store in the fridge until ready to serve.
Nutrition information:
Calories per serving: 57; Carbohydrates:14.1 g; Protein: 1.8g; Fat: 0.2g; Fiber: 2.4g

Chicken Feet Stock

Serves: 8
Preparation Time: 2 minutes
Cooking Time: 60 minutes
Ingredients

- 1 ½ pound chicken feet, cleaned and rinsed
- 8 cups water

Instructions
1. Place all ingredients in the Instant Pot.
2. Close the lid and press the Manual button.
3. Adjust the cooking time to 60 minutes
4. Do natural pressure release.
5. Run the stock through a sieve and discard the solids.
6. Place in mason jars and store in the fridge until ready to serve.

Nutrition information:
Calories per serving: 183; Carbohydrates:0 g; Protein: 16.5g; Fat: 12.4g; Fiber: 0g

Vegan Beef Stock

Serves: 8
Preparation Time:3 minutes
Cooking Time: 25 minutes

Ingredients
- 8 ounces mushrooms, diced
- 2 onions, diced
- 4 stalks of celery, diced
- 3 carrots, peeled and chopped
- ½ cup red wine
- ¼ cup soy sauce
- 4 cloves of garlic
- 2 tablespoons tomato paste
- 1 tablespoon miso paste
- ½ tablespoon balsamic vinegar
- 1 teaspoon black peppercorn
- 1 bay leaf

Instructions
1. Place all ingredients in the Instant Pot.
2. Close the lid and press the Manual button.
3. Adjust the cooking time to 40 minutes
4. Do natural pressure release.
5. Run the stock through a sieve and discard the solids.
6. Place in mason jars and store in the fridge until ready to serve.

Nutrition information:
Calories per serving: 142; Carbohydrates: 30.4g; Protein: 4.3g; Fat: 1.9g; Fiber: 5g

Instant Pot Ham Bone Broth

Serves: 8
Preparation Time: 3 minutes
Cooking Time: 45 minutes

Ingredients
- 1 leftover ham bone
- 8 cups water
- Salt

Instructions
1. Place all ingredients in the Instant Pot.
2. Close the lid and press the Manual button.
3. Adjust the cooking time to 45 minutes
4. Do natural pressure release.
5. Run the stock through a sieve and discard the solids.
6. Place in mason jars and store in the fridge until ready to serve.

Nutrition information:
Calories per serving:46; Carbohydrates: 1.1g; Protein: 4.7g; Fat: 2.4g; Fiber: 0.4g

10-Minute Mushroom Broth

Serves: 8
Preparation Time: 3 minutes
Cooking Time: 10 minutes

Ingredients
- 8 cups water
- ½ cup porcini mushrooms, fresh
- 6 cloves of garlic, crushed
- Salt and pepper
- 1 sprig of thyme

Instructions
1. Place all ingredients in the Instant Pot.
2. Close the lid and press the Manual button.
3. Adjust the cooking time to 10 minutes
4. Do natural pressure release.
5. Run the stock through a sieve and discard the solids.
6. Place in mason jars and store in the fridge until ready to serve.

Nutrition information:
Calories per serving: 7; Carbohydrates: 1.5g; Protein: 0.4g; Fat: 0.01g; Fiber: 0.2g

Chinese Master Stock

Serves: 2
Preparation Time: 3 minutes
Cooking Time: 15 minutes

Ingredients
- 1 cup water
- ½ cup Shaoxing wine
- 3 tablespoons light soy sauce
- 3 tablespoons dark soy sauce
- 1 tablespoon sugar
- 1 teaspoon sesame oil

Instructions
1. Place all ingredients in the Instant Pot.
2. Close the lid and press the Manual button.
3. Adjust the cooking time to 15 minutes
4. Do natural pressure release.
5. Run the stock through a sieve and discard the solids.
6. Place in mason jars and store in the fridge until ready to serve.

Nutrition information:
Calories per serving: 63; Carbohydrates: 7.1g; Protein: 4.5g; Fat: 2.4g; Fiber: 0.3g

Vegan Chicken Stock

Serves: 8
Preparation Time:3 minutes
Cooking Time: 40 minutes

Ingredients
- 1-ounce dried shiitake mushrooms, soaked then rinsed

- 2 cups hot water
- 2 onions, diced
- 3 stalks of celery, chopped
- 2 carrots, chopped
- 3 cloves of garlic, minced
- ½ cup nutritional yeast
- 1 tablespoon miso paste
- 1 teaspoon poultry seasoning
- 8 cups water
- 1 bay leaf
- 2 sprigs thyme
- 1 teaspoon black peppercorns

Instructions
1. Place all ingredients in the Instant Pot.
2. Close the lid and press the Manual button.
3. Adjust the cooking time to 40 minutes
4. Do natural pressure release.
5. Run the stock through a sieve and discard the solids.
6. Place in mason jars and store in the fridge until ready to serve.

Nutrition information:
Calories per serving: 60; Carbohydrates: 9.5g; Protein: 5.2g; Fat: 0.4g; Fiber: 2.4g

Browned Chicken Broth

Serves: 8
Preparation Time: 3 minutes
Cooking Time: 45 minutes

Ingredients
- 3 pounds chicken backs and necks
- 1 onion, halved
- 2 heads of garlic, crushed
- 4 ounces baby carrots, chopped
- 1 stalk of celery, chopped
- 1 teaspoon peppercorns
- 2 bay leaves
- 8 cups

Instructions
1. Press the Sauté button on the Instant Pot.
2. Place the chicken backs and neck and sauté until the meat has turned brown.
3. Add the onion and garlic until fragrant.
4. Place the rest of the ingredients in the Instant Pot.
5. Close the lid and press the Manual button.
6. Adjust the cooking time to 45 minutes
7. Do natural pressure release.
8. Run the stock through a sieve and discard the solids.
9. Place in mason jars and store in the fridge until ready to serve.

Nutrition information:
Calories per serving:183; Carbohydrates:2.5 g; Protein: 14.8g; Fat: 12.6g; Fiber: 0.7g

Classic Chicken Bone Broth

Serves: 8
Preparation Time: 3 minutes
Cooking Time: 60 minutes
Ingredients
- 2-pound raw chicken bones
- 2 carrots, chopped
- 2 stalks of celery, chopped
- 1 onion, chopped
- 3 cloves of garlic, crushed
- 2 teaspoons salt
- 2 tablespoons apple cider vinegar
- 8 cups water

Instructions
1. Place all ingredients in the Instant Pot.
2. Close the lid and press the Manual button.
3. Adjust the cooking time to 60 minutes
4. Do natural pressure release.
5. Run the stock through a sieve and discard the solids.
6. Place in mason jars and store in the fridge until ready to serve.

Nutrition information:
Calories per serving: 142; Carbohydrates: 3.6g; Protein: 23.4g; Fat: 3.1g; Fiber: 0.8g

Leftover Turkey Carcass Soup

Serves: 8
Preparation Time: 3 minutes
Cooking Time: 60 minutes

Ingredients
- Carcass from 1 roasted turkey, preferably leftover from Thanksgiving
- 1 onion, peeled
- 1 stalk celery, chopped
- 1 carrot, chopped
- 2 bay leaves
- 8 cups water

Instructions
1. Place all ingredients in the Instant Pot.
2. Close the lid and press the Manual button.
3. Adjust the cooking time to 60 minutes
4. Do natural pressure release.
5. Run the stock through a sieve and discard the solids.
6. Place in mason jars and store in the fridge until ready to serve.

Nutrition information:
Calories per serving: 123; Carbohydrates: 2.1g; Protein: 7.8g; Fat: 9.1g; Fiber: 0.5g

3-Ingredient Bone Broth

Serves: 8
Preparation Time: 3 minutes
Cooking Time:60 minutes

Ingredients
- 1 whole chicken bones
- 1 tablespoon salt
- ¼ cup apple cider vinegar
- 8 cups water

Instructions
1. Place all ingredients in the Instant Pot.
2. Close the lid and press the Manual button.
3. Adjust the cooking time to 60 minutes
4. Do natural pressure release.

5. Run the stock through a sieve and discard the solids.
6. Place in mason jars and store in the fridge until ready to serve.
Nutrition information:
Calories per serving: 136; Carbohydrates: 0.9g; Protein: 24.5g; Fat: 3.3g; Fiber:0g

Easy Savory Turkey Stock

Serves: 6
Preparation Time: 3 minutes
Cooking Time: 60 minutes
Ingredients
- 1-pound turkey bones
- 1 turkey neck
- 1 package turkey giblets
- 2 carrots, unpeeled and chopped
- 3 stalks of celery, chopped
- 1 onion, halved
- 1 bulb garlic, crushed
- 2 sprigs of sage
- 8 cups water

Instructions
1. Place all ingredients in the Instant Pot.
2. Close the lid and press the Manual button.
3. Adjust the cooking time to 60 minutes
4. Do natural pressure release.
5. Run the stock through a sieve and discard the solids.
6. Place in mason jars and store in the fridge until ready to serve.

Nutrition information:
Calories per serving:184; Carbohydrates:3.9 g; Protein: 28.1g; Fat: 5.4g; Fiber: 1g

Classic Beef Bone Broth

Serves: 8
Preparation Time: 3 minutes
Cooking Time: 1 hour and 30 minutes
Ingredients
- 4 pounds beef bones
- 1 carrots, unpeeled and chopped
- 1 onion, quartered
- 1 head garlic, minced
- 3 stalks celery, chopped
- 2 bay leaves
- 2 tablespoons black peppercorns
- 1 tablespoon apple cider vinegar
- 10 cups water

Instructions
1. Place all ingredients in the Instant Pot.
2. Close the lid and press the Manual button.
3. Adjust the cooking time to 1 hour and 30 minutes
4. Do natural pressure release.
5. Run the stock through a sieve and discard the solids.
6. Place in mason jars and store in fridge until ready to serve.

Nutrition information:
Calories per serving: 252; Carbohydrates: 2.6g; Protein: 31.8g; Fat: 11.8g; Fiber: 0.6g

Soups, Stews, and Chilies Recipes

Cuban Black Bean Soup

Serves: 6
Preparation Time: 5 minutes
Cooking Time: 50 minutes
Ingredients
- 2 tablespoons olive oil
- 1 onion, chopped
- 5 cloves of garlic, minced
- 1 red bell pepper, chopped
- 1 bay leaf
- 1 teaspoon ground cumin
- 2 teaspoons ground oregano
- ½ cup red wine
- 4 cups water
- 2 tablespoons sherry vinegar
- 1-pound dried black beans, soaked overnight
- Salt and pepper

Instructions
1. Press the Sauté button on the Instant Pot.
2. Heat the oil and sauté the onions and garlic until fragrant.
3. Stir in the bell pepper, bay leaf, cumin, and oregano. Stir for another minute.
4. Pour in the red wine, water, sherry vinegar, and beans. Season with salt and pepper to taste.
5. Close the lid and press the Bean/Chili button.
6. Adjust the cooking time to 50 minutes.
7. Do natural pressure release.

Nutrition information:
Calories per serving: 304; Carbohydrates: 51.6g; Protein: 17g; Fat: 5.7g; Fiber: 12.5g

Garden Harvest Soup

Serves: 8
Preparation Time: 3 minutes
Cooking Time: 10 minutes
Ingredients
- 6 cups bone broth
- 10 cup packaged vegetables of your choice
- 1 teaspoon parsley
- 1 teaspoon basil
- 1 teaspoon thyme
- 1 teaspoon rosemary
- 1 can crushed tomatoes
- Salt and pepper to taste

Instructions
1. Place all ingredients in the Instant Pot.
2. Close the lid and press the Manual button.
3. Adjust the cooking time to 10 minutes.
4. Do natural pressure release.

Nutrition information:
Calories per serving: 439; Carbohydrates: 32.5g; Protein: 45.7g; Fat: 12.9g; Fiber: 10.6g

Whole Food Minestrone Soup

Serves: 6
Preparation Time: 5 minutes
Cooking Time: 10 minutes
Ingredients
- 2 tablespoons olive oil
- 1 onion, diced
- 3 cloves of garlic, minced
- 2 stalks of celery, diced
- 1 carrot, diced
- 1 teaspoon dried basil
- 1 teaspoon dried oregano
- Salt and pepper to taste
- 1 can crushed tomatoes
- 1 can white cannellini beans, rinsed
- 1 bay leaf
- 4 cups bone broth
- 1 cup elbow pasta
- 1 cup kale leaves, chopped
- 1/3 cup parmesan cheese, grated

Instructions
1. Press the Sauté button on the Instant Pot.
2. Heat the oil and sauté the onions and garlic until fragrant.
3. Stir in the celery, carrots, basil, and oregano. Season with salt and pepper to taste
4. Add the tomatoes, beans, bay leaf. Pour in the bone broth.
5. Stir in the elbow pasta.
6. Close the lid and press the Manual button.
7. Adjust the cooking time to 10 minutes.
8. Do natural pressure release.
9. Once the lid is open, add the kale leaves and parmesan cheese.

Nutrition information:
Calories per serving: 143; Carbohydrates: 13.5g; Protein: 6.4g; Fat: 7.3g; Fiber: 2.8g

Instant Pot Football Chili

Serves: 6
Preparation Time: 5 minutes
Cooking Time: 15 minutes
Ingredients
- 2 pounds ground beef
- 2 cups corn kernels
- 2 cups tomatoes, chopped
- 2 packets of taco seasoning
- 1 can red beans, rinsed and drained
- 1 can pinto beans, rinsed and drained
- 1 can black beans, rinsed and drained
- 2 cans beef stock
- Salt and pepper

Instructions
1. Press the Sauté button on the Instant Pot.
2. Put the ground beef and sauté the beef for three minutes.
3. Pour in the rest of the ingredients.
4. Close the lid and press the Chili/Bean button.
5. Adjust the cooking time to 15 minutes.
6. Do natural pressure release.
7. Serve on taco shells or with sour cream and avocado slices.

Nutrition information:
Calories per serving: 663; Carbohydrates: 50.8g; Protein: 55.3g; Fat: 26.7g; Fiber: 12g

Beef Borscht Soup

Serves: 6
Preparation Time: 5 minutes

Cooking Time: 20 minutes
Ingredients
- 2 pounds ground beef
- 3 beets, peeled and diced
- 3 stalks of celery, diced
- 2 large carrots, diced
- 2 cloves of garlic, diced
- 1 onion, diced
- 3 cups shredded cabbage
- 6 cups beef stock
- 1 bay leaf
- ½ tablespoon thyme
- Salt and pepper

Instructions
1. Press the Sauté button on the Instant Pot.
2. Sauté the beef for 5 minutes until slightly golden.
3. Add all the rest of the ingredients in the Instant Pot.
4. Close the lid and press the Manual button.
5. Adjust the cooking time to 15 minutes.
6. Do natural pressure release.

Nutrition information:
Calories per serving: 477; Carbohydrates: 17.7g; Protein: 44.5g; Fat: 24.9g; Fiber: 3.2g

Chicken and Sweet Potato Chipotle Soup

Serves: 8
Preparation Time: 3 minutes
Cooking Time: 10 minutes
Ingredients
- 2 tablespoons coconut oil
- 1 onion, chopped
- 3 cloves of garlic, minced
- 1 teaspoon chipotle seasoning
- ½ taco seasoning
- 6 cups sweet potatoes, peeled and chopped
- 6 cups chicken soup
- 3 cans cannellini beans
- 4 cups cooked chicken, shredded
- salt and pepper

Instructions
1. Press the Sauté button on the Instant Pot.
2. Heat the oil and sauté the onion and garlic until fragrant.
3. Add the chipotle and taco seasonings.
4. Stir in the sweet potatoes, chicken soup, cannellini beans, and chicken strips.
5. Season with salt and pepper to taste.
6. Close the lid and press the Manual button.
7. Adjust the cooking time to 7 minutes.
8. Do natural pressure release.

Nutrition information:
Calories per serving: 401; Carbohydrates: 14.6g; Protein: 21.6g; Fat: 28.7g; Fiber: 2.6g

Swiss Chard Stem Soup

Serves: 6
Preparation Time: 3 minutes
Cooking Time: 4 minutes
Ingredients
- 8 cups Swiss Chard stems, diced
- 3 leeks, chopped
- 1 celeriac, peeled and diced
- 1 potato, peeled and diced
- 1 ½ cups chicken stock
- 1 cup coconut milk
- Salt and pepper to taste

Instructions
1. Place all ingredients in the Instant Pot.
2. Give a good stir to combine everything.
3. Close the lid and press the Manual button.
4. Adjust the cooking time to 4 minutes.
5. Do natural pressure release.

Nutrition information:
Calories per serving: 200; Carbohydrates: 23.9g; Protein: 5.4g; Fat: 10.6g; Fiber: 3.9g

Instant Pot Chicken Tortilla Soup

Serves: 4
Preparation Time: 5 minutes
Cooking Time: 12 minutes
Ingredients
- 1 tablespoon olive oil
- 1 onion, chopped
- 2 cloves of garlic, minced
- 2 tablespoons fresh cilantro, chopped
- 1 large ripe tomato, chopped
- 1 can black beans, drained and rinsed
- 1 cup frozen corn
- 4 cups chicken broth
- 2 teaspoons chili powder
- 1 teaspoon cumin powder
- 1 bay leaf
- Salt and pepper to taste
- 3 cooked chicken breasts, shredded
- 2 cooked corn tortillas, crumbled

Instructions
1. Press the Sauté button on the Instant Pot.
2. Heat the olive oil and sauté the onion and garlic until fragrant.
3. Stir in the cilantro, tomatoes, black beans, corn, and chicken broth.
4. Season with chili powder, cumin, bay leaf, salt, and pepper.
5. Add the chicken last.
6. Close the lid and press the Soup button.
7. Adjust the cooking time to 6 minutes.
8. Do quick pressure release.
9. Sprinkle with cooked corn tortillas on top.

Nutrition information:
Calories per serving: 840; Carbohydrates: 43.5g; Protein: 102.8g; Fat: 26.4g; Fiber: 10.8g

Instant Pot Cheddar, Broccoli, And Potato Soup

Serves: 6
Preparation Time: 5 minutes
Cooking Time: 7 minutes
Ingredients
- 2 tablespoons butter
- 2 cloves of garlic, minced
- 1 broccoli head, cut into florets
- 2 pounds Yukon Gold potatoes, peeled and quartered
- 4 cups chicken broth
- Salt and pepper to taste
- 1 cup cheddar cheese, grated

- 6 slices of bacon, fried and crumbled

Instructions
1. Press the Sauté button on the Instant Pot.
2. Heat the butter and sauté the garlic until fragrant.
3. Stir in the broccoli florets, potatoes, and chicken broth
4. Season with salt and pepper to taste.
5. Sprinkle with cheese on top.
6. Close the lid and press the Soup button.
7. Adjust the cooking time to 7 minutes.
8. Do quick pressure release.
9. Sprinkle with bacon bits on top.

Nutrition information:
Calories per serving:598; Carbohydrates: 34.4g; Protein: 47.7g; Fat: 29.5g; Fiber: 3.9g

Instant Pot Lasagna Soup

Serves: 7
Preparation Time: 3 minutes
Cooking Time: 10 minutes

Ingredients
- 2 tablespoons olive oil
- 1 onion, chopped
- ½ green pepper, chopped
- 2 carrots, peeled and chopped
- 1 small zucchini, chopped
- 1 can diced tomatoes
- 4 cups vegetable stock
- 2 cups water
- ½ box of lasagna noodles, broken into small pieces
- ½ teaspoon onion powder
- 1 teaspoon oregano
- Salt and pepper

Instructions
1. Press the Sauté button on the Instant Pot.
2. Heat the oil and sauté the onion until fragrant.
3. Stir in the rest of the ingredients.
4. Close the lid and press the Soup button.
5. Adjust the cooking time to 10 minutes.
6. Do quick pressure release.

Nutrition information:
Calories per serving:154; Carbohydrates: 25.6g; Protein: 3.8g; Fat: 4.2g; Fiber: 1.6g

Chicken Faux Pho

Serves: 3
Preparation Time: 5 minutes
Cooking Time: 30 minutes

Ingredients
- 2 onions, quartered
- 1 thumb-size ginger, peeled and chopped
- 1 tablespoon coriander seeds
- 1 teaspoon green cardamom pods
- 1 black cardamom pod
- 1 cinnamon stick
- 4 cloves
- 1 lemongrass stalk, trimmed
- 6 cups chicken stock
- ¼ cup fish sauce
- 4 chicken pieces, bone-in, and skin intact
- 1 cup cilantro
- Salt to taste
- 1 head bok choy, chopped
- Lime wedges
- Fresh basil leaves
- Mung bean sprouts
- ¼ onion, sliced

Instructions
1. Press the Sauté button on the Instant Pot.
2. Place the onions, ginger, coriander seeds, cardamom pods, cinnamon stick, cloves, and lemongrass inside. Allow the surface of the spices to brown for a few minutes.
3. Pour in the chicken stock.
4. Close the lid and press the Soup button. Adjust the cooking time to 15 minutes.
5. Do quick pressure release.
6. Take out the spices from the soup base and add in the fish sauce, chicken, and cilantro. Season with salt and pepper to taste.
7. Close the lid and press the Soup button. Adjust the cooking time to 10 minutes.
8. Do quick pressure release.
9. Press the Sauté button and add the bok choy. Allow simmering until the veggies have wilted.
10. Serve with lime wedges, basil leaves, mung bean sprouts and sliced onions.

Nutrition information:
Calories per serving: 448; Carbohydrates: 29.2g; Protein: 42.2g; Fat: 21.8g; Fiber: 2.8g

Ethiopian Spinach and Lentil Soup

Serves: 6
Preparation Time: 5 minutes
Cooking Time: 60 minutes

Ingredients
- 2 tablespoons butter
- 1 tablespoon olive oil
- 1 onion, finely chopped
- 1 teaspoon garlic powder
- 2 teaspoons ground coriander
- ½ teaspoon cinnamon powder
- ½ teaspoon turmeric powder
- ¼ teaspoon clove powder
- ¼ teaspoon cayenne pepper
- ¼ teaspoon cardamom powder
- ¼ teaspoon nutmeg, grated
- 2 cups lentils, soaked overnight then rinsed
- 8 cups water
- Salt and pepper
- 2 cups spinach leaves, chopped
- 4 tablespoons lemon juice

Instructions
1. Press the Sauté button on the Instant Pot and heat the butter and olive oil.
2. Sauté the onion, garlic powder, coriander, cinnamon, turmeric, clove, cayenne pepper, cardamom, and nutmeg until fragrant.
3. Add the lentils and season with salt and pepper to taste.
4. Close the lid and press the Manual button.
5. Adjust the cooking time to 60 minutes or until the beans are soft.
6. Do quick pressure release.
7. Once the lid is off, press the Sauté button and add the spinach leaves and lemon juice. Simmer until the leaves have wilted.

Nutrition information:
Calories per serving: 113; Carbohydrates: 11.9g;
Protein: 4.7g; Fat: 6.7g; Fiber:2.7g

Mexican Meatball Soup

Serves: 6
Preparation Time: 5 minutes
Cooking Time: 20 minutes
Ingredients
- 1 tablespoon olive oil
- 2 cloves of garlic, minced
- 1 onion, chopped
- 1 package prepared meatballs
- 1 green bell pepper, chopped
- 1 tablespoon oregano
- ½ teaspoon cumin
- 1 cup carrots, chopped finely
- 1 can diced tomatoes
- Salt and pepper to taste
- 1 egg, lightly beaten

Instructions
1. Press the Sauté button on the Instant Pot.
2. Heat the olive oil and sauté the garlic and onions until fragrant.
3. Add the meatballs and brown the sides for a few minutes.
4. Stir in the rest of the ingredients except for the eggs.
5. Close the lid and press the Soup button.
6. Adjust the cooking time to 15 minutes.
7. Do quick pressure release.
8. Once the lid is open, press the Sauté button.
9. Stir in the beaten egg and allow to cook for 3 minutes.

Nutrition information:
Calories per serving: 398; Carbohydrates: 19.9g;
Protein: 37.5g; Fat:19.1g; Fiber: 9.4g

Hearty and Creamy Broccoli Soup

Serves: 6
Preparation Time: 5 minutes
Cooking Time: 10 minutes
Ingredients
- 1 tablespoon vegetable oil
- 1 onion, chopped
- 3 cloves of garlic, diced
- 1 can mushroom broth
- 1 cup water
- 1 cup almond milk, unsweetened
- 1 large broccoli head, cut into florets
- 1 Yukon Gold potato, cut into chunks
- 3 teaspoons nutritional yeasts
- 2 tablespoons soy sauce
- Salt and pepper to taste

Instructions
1. Press the Sauté button on the Instant Pot.
2. Heat the oil.
3. Sauté the onion and garlic until fragrant.
4. Add in the rest of the ingredients.
5. Close the lid and press the Manual button.
6. Adjust the cooking time to 7 minutes.
7. Do natural pressure release.

Nutrition information:
Calories per serving: 138; Carbohydrates: 21.3g;
Protein: 3.7g; Fat: 4.6g; Fiber:2.3g

Butternut and Cauliflower Stew

Serves: 6
Preparation Time: 5 minutes
Cooking Time: 15 minutes
Ingredients
- 1 teaspoon olive oil
- 1 onion, chopped
- 3 cloves of garlic, minced
- 1 cauliflower head, cut into florets
- 1-pound butternut squash, seeded and chopped
- 2 cups vegetable broth
- 1 teaspoon paprika
- 1 teaspoon dried thyme
- ½ teaspoon red pepper flakes
- Salt to taste
- ½ cup whole milk

Instructions
1. Press the Sauté button on the Instant Pot.
2. Pour in the oil and sauté the onion and garlic until fragrant.
3. Add the rest of the ingredients.
4. Close the lid and press the Soup button.
5. Adjust the cooking time to 12 minutes.
6. Do natural pressure release.
7. Top with bacon bits or grated parmesan cheese if desired.

Nutrition information:
Calories per serving:244; Carbohydrates: 17.6g;
Protein: 2.6g; Fat: 1.7g; Fiber: 2.9g

Instant Pot Cheeseburger Soup

Serves: 5
Preparation Time: 5 minutes
Cooking Time: 15 minutes
Ingredients
- 1-pound lean ground beef
- ½ cup carrots, shredded
- 2 cups potatoes, peeled and cubed
- 3 cups beef broth
- 1 can diced tomatoes
- 2 cups heavy cream
- 1 cup cheddar cheese, grated
- 1 onion, diced

Instructions
1. Press the Sauté button on the Instant Pot.
2. Add the beef and cook until brown and has slightly rendered its fat. Drain the grease.
3. Pour in the rest of the ingredients and give a good stir.
4. Close the lid and press the Soup button.
5. Adjust the cooking time to 15 minutes.
6. Do natural pressure release.

Nutrition information:
Calories per serving:579; Carbohydrates: 34.7 g;
Protein: 34.5g; Fat: 33.2g; Fiber: 2.9g

Instant Pot Zuppa Toscana

Serves: 6
Preparation Time: 5 minutes
Cooking Time: 20 minutes

Ingredients
- 2 tablespoons olive oil
- 1-pound Italian sausages, chopped
- 1 onion, diced
- 4 cloves of garlic, minced
- 3 large russet potatoes, unpeeled and sliced thickly
- 6 cups chicken broth
- ¼ cup water
- Salt and pepper
- 2 cups kale, chopped
- ¾ cup heavy cream

Instructions
1. Press the Sauté button on the Instant Pot.
2. Sauté the Italian sausages, onions, and garlic for a few minutes until the sausages have turned slightly golden.
3. Stir in the potatoes, chicken broth, and water. Season with salt and pepper to taste.
4. Close the lid and press the Manual button.
5. Adjust the cooking time to 20 minutes.
6. Do quick pressure release.
7. Once the lid is open, press the Sauté button and add the kale and heavy cream until.
8. Allow simmering for 3 minutes.
9. Serve.

Nutrition information:
Calories per serving: 553; Carbohydrates: 40.7g; Protein: 20.5g; Fat: 35.4g; Fiber:3.9g

Creamy Thai Coconut Chicken Soup

Serves: 4
Preparation Time: 5 minutes
Cooking Time: 20 minutes

Ingredients
- 2 tablespoons oil
- 1 onion, quartered
- 2 pounds chicken breasts, skin and bones removed
- 2 tablespoons Thai red curry paste
- 1 red bell pepper, cut into strips
- 6 slices galangal or ginger
- 6 kaffir lime leaves
- 3 cups chicken broth
- 2 tablespoons fish sauce
- 1 tablespoon sugar
- ¾ cup coconut milk
- 2 ½ tablespoons lime juice
- Cilantro leaves for serving

Instructions
1. Press the Sauté button on the Instant Pot.
2. Heat the oil and sauté the onion and chicken. Turn the chicken constantly until slightly golden.
3. Add the red curry paste, bell pepper, galangal, and kaffir limes.
4. After 30 seconds, add the chicken broth, fish sauce, and sugar.
5. Close the lid and press the Manual button.
6. Adjust the cooking button to 15 minutes.
7. Do quick pressure release.
8. Once the lid is open, press the Sauté button and add the coconut milk and lime juice.
9. Allow simmering for 5 more minutes.
10. Serve with cilantro leaves.

Nutrition information:
Calories per serving: 624; Carbohydrates: 17.8g; Protein: 52.6g; Fat: 39.1g; Fiber: 3.7g

Red Lentil Chili

Serves: 10
Preparation Time: 5 minutes
Cooking Time: 60 minutes

Ingredients
- 1-pound red lentils, soaked overnight then rinsed
- 7 cups water
- 2 cans crushed tomatoes
- 2 tablespoons tomato paste
- 2 cups red bell peppers, chopped
- ¼ cup Medjool dates, pitted and chopped
- 8 cloves of garlic, minced
- 4 tablespoons apple cider vinegar
- 1 ½ tablespoons parsley flaked
- 1 ½ tablespoons oregano
- 1 ½ tablespoons chili powder
- Salt and pepper

Instructions
1. Place all ingredients in the Instant Pot.
2. Give a good stir.
3. Close the lid and press the Manual button.
4. Adjust the cooking time to 60 minutes.
5. Do natural pressure release.

Nutrition information:
Calories per serving: 188; Carbohydrates:34.4 g; Protein: 11.9g; Fat: 1.3g; Fiber:6.5 g

Instant Pot Pork Vindaloo

Serves: 8
Preparation Time: 5 minutes
Cooking Time: 25 minutes

Ingredients
- ¼ cup olive oil
- 1 onion, chopped
- 4 cloves of garlic, minced
- 3 pounds pork shoulder, cubed
- 1 thumb-sized ginger, peeled and grated
- 2 tablespoons Madras or vindaloo curry seasoning
- 1 teaspoon hot paprika
- ½ teaspoon ground turmeric
- 1/3 cup champagne vinegar
- 1 can diced tomatoes
- 1 cup chicken stock
- Salt and pepper

Instructions
1. Press the Sauté button on the Instant Pot.
2. Heat the oil and sauté the onion and garlic.
3. Stir in the pork shoulder pieces and continue cooking until slightly browned.
4. Add the rest of the ingredients.
5. Scrape the bottom of the pot to remove the browning.
6. Close the lid and press the Manual button.
7. Adjust the cooking time to 20 minutes.
8. Do natural pressure release.

Nutrition information:
Calories per serving:547; Carbohydrates: 5.5g; Protein: 44.2g; Fat: 37.5g; Fiber:1.8 g

Instant Pot Goat Stew

Serves: 3
Preparation Time: 5 minutes
Cooking Time: 40 minutes
Ingredients
- 2 tablespoons olive oil
- 1 onion, chopped
- 3 cloves of garlic, minced
- 1 tablespoon cumin seeds
- ½ pound goat meat, chopped
- 1 stalk of celery, chopped
- 1 carrot, peeled and chunked
- ¼ cup tomato paste
- A dash of balsamic vinegar
- 1 cup chicken stock
- ½ cup water
- 1 teaspoon dried rosemary leaves
- Salt and pepper

Instructions
1. Press the Sauté button on the Instant Pot.
2. Heat the oil and sauté the onion and garlic. Stir in the cumin seeds.
3. Stir in the goat meat and brown all sides for a few minutes.
4. Add the celery, carrots, tomato paste, and balsamic vinegar.
5. Pour in the chicken stock, water, and rosemary. Season with salt and pepper.
6. Close the lid and press the Manual button.
7. Adjust the cooking time to 60 minutes.
8. Do natural pressure release.

Nutrition information:
Calories per serving: 304; Carbohydrates: 12g; Protein: 36.3g; Fat:11.5g; Fiber: 2.6g

Instant Pot Kimchi Stew (Korean Kimchi Jjigae)

Serves: 6
Preparation Time: 5 minutes
Cooking Time: 25 minutes
Ingredients
- 1 tablespoon oil
- 1 onion, sliced
- 1-pound pork belly, cut into chunks
- 3 cups sour Korean kimchi cabbage, chopped
- ¼ cup kimchi juice
- 4 cups water
- 1 tablespoon sugar
- Package firm tofu
- 3 green onions, chopped
- 1 teaspoon sesame oil
- 2 tablespoons sesame seeds, toasted

Instructions
1. Press the Sauté button on the Instant Pot.
2. Heat the oil and sauté the onions until fragrant.
3. Stir in the pork belly slices. Stir until slightly golden.
4. Add the kimchi, kimchi juice, and water. Season with sugar.
5. Season with salt if needed.
6. Close the lid and press the Manual button.
7. Adjust the cooking time to 20 minutes.
8. Do quick pressure release.
9. Once the lid is open, press the Sauté button.
10. Add in the firm tofu and allow to simmer for 5 minutes.
11. Garnish with green onions, a drizzle of sesame oil, and sesame seeds.

Nutrition information:
Calories per serving: 475; Carbohydrates: 8.63g; Protein: 8.99g; Fat: 45.41g; Fiber: 2g

Puchero A La Valencia (Spanish Stew)

Serves: 8
Preparation Time: 2 minutes
Cooking Time: 30 minutes
Ingredients
- 1 daikon radish, peeled and sliced thickly
- 1 rutabaga, peeled and sliced thickly
- 2 carrots, peeled and cut into chunks
- 2 stalks of celery, chopped
- 1 bunch artichoke hearts, trimmed and sliced
- 2 large beef bones
- ¼ cup chicken breasts, cut into chunks
- 1-pound beef stew meat, cut into chunks
- A pinch of saffron
- 1 can garbanzos beans, drained and rinsed
- 4 cups water

Instructions
1. Place all ingredients in the Instant Pot.
2. Close the lid and press the Manual button.
3. Adjust the cooking time to 30 minutes.
4. Do natural pressure release.

Nutrition information:
Calories per serving: 469; Carbohydrates: 8.4g; Protein: 8.6g; Fat: 44.9g; Fiber: 1.9g

Instant Pot Ham and Potato Soup

Serves: 5
Preparation Time: 5 minutes
Cooking Time: 30 minutes
Ingredients
- 2 tablespoons butter
- 1 onion, diced
- 8 cloves of garlic, minced
- 2 pounds Yukon Gold potatoes, cut into small chunks
- 4 cups chicken broth
- A dash of cayenne pepper
- ½ cup cheddar cheese, grated
- 1 cup cooked ham, diced
- Salt and pepper
- 2 tablespoons fried bacon bits

Instructions
1. Press the Sauté button on the Instant Pot.
2. Heat the butter and sauté the onions and garlic until fragrant.
3. Stir in the potatoes and cook for 3 minutes.
4. Pour in the broth, cayenne pepper, cheese, and cooked ham. Season with salt and pepper to taste.
5. Close the lid and press the Manual button.
6. Adjust the cooking time to 25 minutes.
7. Do quick pressure release.
8. Open the lid and garnish with bacon bits on top.

Nutrition information:
Calories per serving: 394; Carbohydrates: 46.7g; Protein: 24.5g; Fat: 13.3g; Fiber:5.1g

Easy Corn Chowder

Serves: 6
Preparation Time: 5 minutes
Cooking Time: 10 minutes
Ingredients
- 1 tablespoon olive oil
- 1 onion, chopped
- 1 red bell pepper, diced
- 1 green bell pepper, diced
- 3 potatoes, cubed
- 4 cups corn kernels
- Salt and pepper
- 4 cups chicken broth
- 3 tablespoons butter
- 1 cup milk + 1 tablespoon flour

Instructions
1. Press the Sauté button on the Instant Pot.
2. Heat the oil and sauté the onions until fragrant.
3. Add the bell peppers, potatoes, and corn kernels. Season with salt and pepper to taste.
4. Pour in the chicken broth.
5. Close the lid and press the Manual button.
6. Adjust the cooking time to 6 minutes.
7. Do quick pressure release.
8. Once the lid is open, press the Sauté button.
9. Stir in the butter and milk mixture.
10. Simmer for 3 minutes or until the sauce has thickened.

Nutrition information:
Calories per serving:580; Carbohydrates: 55.8g; Protein: 42.9g; Fat: 21.6g; Fiber: 7.3g

Beans and Tomato Stew

Serves: 6
Preparation Time: 5 minutes
Cooking Time: 60 minutes
Ingredients
- 1 cup dried chickpeas, soaked overnight then drained
- 1 cup dried white beans, soaked overnight then drained
- 2 tablespoons olive oil
- 1 onion, chopped
- 2 stalks of celery, chopped
- 1 ½ teaspoon dried dill
- 1 ½ teaspoons ground cinnamon
- 1 ½ tablespoons mild paprika
- 1 can diced tomatoes
- 2 tablespoons tomato paste
- 2 ¾ cups vegetable broth
- Salt and pepper

Instructions
1. Place all ingredients in the Instant Pot.
2. Stir to combine everything.
3. Close the lid and press the Manual button.
4. Adjust the cooking time to 60 minutes.
5. Do quick pressure release.

Nutrition information:
Calories per serving:312; Carbohydrates: 49.1g; Protein: 15.8g; Fat: 7.3g; Fiber: 11.6g

African Peanut Butter Beef Stew

Serves: 6
Preparation Time: 5 minutes
Cooking Time: 35 minutes
Ingredients
- 1 tablespoon oil
- 1 onion, diced
- 4 cloves of garlic, minced
- 2 pounds beef stew meat, cut into chunks
- 1 teaspoon paprika
- 1 teaspoon ground coriander
- 1 teaspoon ground cumin
- ½ teaspoon nutmeg
- ¼ teaspoon fenugreek powder
- Salt and pepper to taste
- 2 tablespoons tomato paste
- 2 cups beef broth
- 1 cup water
- ¾ cup creamy peanut butter
- 1 thumb-size ginger, sliced
- ½ cups peanuts, roasted

Instructions
1. Press the Sauté button on the Instant Pot.
2. Heat the oil and sauté the onions and garlic until fragrant.
3. Add in the beef stew meat and season with paprika, coriander, cumin, nutmeg and fenugreek powder. Stir in salt and pepper to taste.
4. Cook for 3 minutes until the beef is slightly golden.
5. Add the tomato paste, broth, water, peanut butter, and ginger.
6. Give a good stir.
7. Close the lid and press the Manual button.
8. Adjust the cooking time to 30 minutes.
9. Do natural pressure release.
10. Once the lid is open, garnish with peanuts.

Nutrition information:
Calories per serving:515; Carbohydrates: 27.8g; Protein: 15.8g; Fat: 40.8g; Fiber: 4.8g

Italian Sausage Stew

Serves: 4
Preparation Time: 5 minutes
Cooking Time: 30 minutes
Ingredients
- 2 tablespoons butter
- ½ pound ground pork
- ½ teaspoon onion powder
- ½ teaspoon garlic powder
- 1 ½ teaspoon basil
- ½ teaspoon thyme
- ¼ teaspoon cumin
- ½ teaspoon marjoram
- ¼ teaspoon cayenne
- 2 carrots, diced
- 2 stalks of celery, chopped
- ½ cup wine
- 1 can diced tomatoes
- 4 cups bone broth
- Salt and pepper
- A handful of kale, chopped
- ½ cup parmesan cheese, grated

Instructions
1. Press the Sauté button on the Instant Pot.

2. Melt the oil and add the ground pork. Stir in the onion powder, garlic powder, basil, thyme, cumin, marjoram, and cayenne.
3. Continue stirring the pork until lightly golden.
4. Stir in the carrots, celery, wine, tomatoes, and bone broth.
5. Season with salt and pepper.
6. Close the lid and press the Manual button.
7. Adjust the cooking time to 25 minutes.
8. Do quick pressure release.
9. Once the lid is open, press the Sauté button and stir in the kale. Simmer until wilted.
10. Sprinkle with parmesan cheese.
Nutrition information:
Calories per serving: 304; Carbohydrates: 8.9g; Protein:21.3g; Fat:19.4 g; Fiber: 2.7g

Enchilada Chicken Stew

Serves: 6
Preparation Time: 5 minutes
Cooking Time: 20 minutes
Ingredients
- 2 tablespoons coconut oil
- 1 onion, chopped
- 3 cloves of garlic, minced
- 2 pounds chicken breasts
- 1 green bell pepper, chopped
- 1 can jalapenos, chopped
- 1 can green chilies, chopped
- 1 can diced tomatoes
- 1 can tomato sauce
- 1 tablespoon cumin
- 1 tablespoon chili powder
- 2 teaspoons dried oregano
- Salt and pepper to taste

Instructions
1. Press the Sauté button on the Instant Pot.
2. Heat the oil and sauté the onion and garlic until fragrant.
3. Add in the chicken breasts and continue stirring until lightly brown.
4. Add the rest of the ingredients
5. Give a good stir.
6. Close the lid and press the Manual button.
7. Adjust the cooking time to 15 minutes.
8. Do natural pressure release.
9. Serve with avocado slices if desired.
Nutrition information:
Calories per serving: 385; Carbohydrates:17.1 g; Protein:34.2 g; Fat: 19.3g; Fiber:5.8 g

Instant Pot Goulash

Serves: 5
Preparation Time: 5 minutes
Cooking Time: 20 minutes
Ingredients
- 1 tablespoon olive oil
- 1 onion, chopped
- 3 cloves of garlic, minced
- 1-pound ground beef
- 2 carrots, chopped
- 3 cups beef broth
- 2 cans tomato sauce
- 2 cans diced tomatoes
- 1 tablespoon Worcestershire sauce
- ½ teaspoon dried thyme
- ½ teaspoon oregano
- 1 cup dry elbow pasta
- Salt and pepper to taste

Instructions
1. Press the Sauté button on the Instant Pot.
2. Heat the oil and sauté the onion and garlic until fragrant.
3. Stir in the ground beef and stir for 3 minutes.
4. Add the rest of the ingredients.
5. Close the lid and press the Manual button.
6. Adjust the cooking time to 15 minutes.
7. Do quick pressure release.
Nutrition information:
Calories per serving:651; Carbohydrates: 81.5g; Protein: 32.3g; Fat: 18.9g; Fiber:18.1g

Instant Pot Carne Guisada

Serves: 5
Preparation Time: 5 minutes
Cooking Time: 35 minutes
Ingredients
- 2 tablespoons olive oil
- 1 onion, chopped
- 3 cloves of garlic, minced
- 1-pound beef stew meat, cut into chunks
- 1 Serrano peppers, minced
- 1 bay leaf
- 1 teaspoon ground cumin
- 1 teaspoon chili powder
- 1 teaspoon paprika
- ½ teaspoon chipotle powder
- ½ teaspoon oregano
- 1 cup beef broth
- ½ cup tomato sauce
- Salt and pepper

Instructions
1. Press the Sauté button on the Instant Pot.
2. Heat the oil and sauté the onion and garlic until fragrant.
3. Stir in the beef and stir for 3 minutes.
4. Add the rest of the ingredients.
5. Close the lid and press the Manual button.
6. Adjust the cooking time to 30 minutes.
7. Do quick pressure release.
Nutrition information:
Calories per serving:189; Carbohydrates: 15.9g; Protein:1.9g; Fat:13.4 g; Fiber: 3.1g

Instant Pot Turkey Chili

Serves: 6
Preparation Time: 5 minutes
Cooking Time: 15 minutes
Ingredients
- 1 tablespoon olive oil
- 1-pound lean ground turkey
- 1 onion, chopped
- 1 tablespoon chili powder
- 2 teaspoons chipotle pepper
- 2 teaspoons ground cumin
- 1 teaspoon garlic powder

- 2 medium sweet potatoes, peeled and sliced thickly
- 1 medium red bell pepper, diced
- 1 can crushed tomatoes
- 2 cans beans, drained and rinsed
- 1 ½ cups chicken broth
- Salt and pepper to taste

Instructions
1. Press the Sauté button on the Instant Pot.
2. Heat the oil and sauté the ground turkey meat.
3. Stir in the onions, chili powder, chipotle pepper, cumin, and garlic powder until fragrant.
4. Add the rest of the ingredients.
5. Scrape the bottom to remove the browning.
6. Close the lid and press the Manual button.
7. Adjust the cooking time to 10 minutes.
8. Do quick pressure release.
9. Serve with cilantro or avocado slices

Nutrition information:
Calories per serving: 346; Carbohydrates: 49g; Protein: 31g; Fat: 4g; Fiber: 14g

Classic Beef Chili

Serves: 6
Preparation Time: 5 minutes
Cooking Time: 20 minutes

Ingredients
- 1-pound ground beef
- 1 onion, diced
- 3 cloves of garlic, minced
- 1 bell pepper, diced
- 1 tablespoon chili powder
- 2/3 tablespoon cumin
- 1 teaspoon ground cumin
- ½ tablespoon brown sugar
- 1 teaspoon hot sauce
- 1/3 cup red wine
- 2 cans kidney beans, undrained
- 1 can diced tomatoes, undrained
- 1 can green chilies, drained
- ¼ cup ketchup
- Salt and pepper

Instructions
1. Press the Sauté button and add in the beef, onions, and garlic.
2. Break the beef and stir for 3 minutes.
3. Add the rest of the ingredients.
4. Give a good stir.
5. Close the lid and press the Manual button.
6. Adjust the cooking time to 15 minutes.
7. Do quick pressure release.
8. Serve with cilantro or avocado slices

Nutrition information:
Calories per serving: 249; Carbohydrates: 22.2g; Protein: 27 g; Fat: 5.5g; Fiber: 6.9g

Instant Pot Chipotle Chili

Serves: 6
Preparation Time: 5 minutes
Cooking Time: 60 minutes

Ingredients
- 1 tablespoon oil
- 1-pound ground beef
- 1 onion, chopped
- 6 cloves of garlic, minced
- ½ teaspoon chipotle chili powder
- 1 tablespoon red chili powder
- 1 teaspoon oregano
- 1 teaspoon cumin powder
- 2 cups tomatoes, chopped
- 1 cup dry kidney beans, soaked overnight and rinsed
- 2 cups chicken broth
- Salt and pepper to taste

Instructions
1. Press the Sauté button and heat the oil.
2. Stir in the ground beef. Break the beef and stir for 3 minutes.
3. Add the onions and garlic until fragrant.
4. Add the rest of the ingredients.
5. Give a good stir.
6. Close the lid and press the Manual button.
7. Adjust the cooking time to 60 minutes.
8. Do quick pressure release.

Nutrition information:
Calories per serving: 405; Carbohydrates: 13.5g; Protein: 40.2g; Fat: 20.6g; Fiber: 3.9g

Instant Pot Cowboy Chili

Serves: 8
Preparation Time: 5 minutes
Cooking Time: 15 minutes

Ingredients
- 1-pound breakfast sausage, chopped
- 1-pound ground beef
- 2 onions, diced
- 2 tablespoons chili powder
- 1 teaspoon garlic powder
- 1 teaspoon onion powder
- ½ teaspoon paprika
- 1 ½ cups tomatoes, chopped
- 1 ½ cups carrots, diced
- 1 cup water
- Salt and pepper

Instructions
1. Press the Sauté button and add the breakfast sausages, ground beef, and onions.
2. Stir for 3 minutes until the meat has rendered some of its fat.
3. Add the rest of the ingredients.
4. Give a good stir.
5. Close the lid and press the Manual button.
6. Adjust the cooking time to 15 minutes.
7. Do quick pressure release.

Nutrition information:
Calories per serving: 312; Carbohydrates: 8.7 g; Protein: 24.7g; Fat: 19.5g; Fiber: 2.6g

Instant Pot Green Chili Stew

Serves: 10
Preparation Time: 5 minutes
Cooking Time: 60 minutes

Ingredients
- 1-pound ground beef
- 1 teaspoon chili powder
- 1 teaspoon ground cumin

- 1 teaspoon garlic powder
- 1 teaspoon onion powder
- 1 onion, diced
- 2 carrots, sliced
- 2 stalks of celery, diced
- 5 cloves of garlic, minced
- 2 cups vegetable broth
- 2 cups water
- 1 teaspoon oregano
- 1 cup dried pinto beans, soaked overnight and rinsed
- 1 can fire-roasted tomatoes
- 1 package Mexico green chilies
- ¼ cup lime juice
- Salt and pepper to taste

Instructions
1. Press the Sauté button on the Instant Pot.
2. Add in the ground beef and season with the chili powder, ground cumin, garlic powder, onion, powder, onions, carrots, celery, and garlic. Mix until well combined and fragrant.
3. Stir in the remaining ingredients.
4. Scrape the bottom of the pot to remove the browning.
5. Close the lid and press the Manual button.
6. Adjust the cooking time to 60 minutes.
7. Do natural pressure release.

Nutrition information:
Calories per serving:202; Carbohydrates: 16.7g; Protein: 16.2g; Fat:7.8g; Fiber: 4g

Texas Beef Chili

Serves: 8
Preparation Time: 5 minutes
Cooking Time: 20 minutes

Ingredients
- 1-pound ground beef
- 1 green bell pepper, seeded and chopped
- 1 onion, diced
- 4 large carrots, chopped finely
- 1 can crushed tomatoes
- 1 teaspoon onion powder
- 1 tablespoon parsley, chopped
- 1 tablespoon Worcestershire sauce
- 4 teaspoons chili powder
- 1 teaspoon paprika
- 1 teaspoon cumin
- 1 teaspoon garlic powder
- Salt and pepper

Instructions
1. Press the Sauté button on the Instant Pot.
2. Add in the ground beef and add in the bell peppers and onions until fragrant.
3. Pour in the rest of the ingredients.
4. Close the lid and press the Manual button.
5. Adjust the cooking time to 15 minutes.
6. Do natural pressure release.

Nutrition information:
Calories per serving: 267; Carbohydrates: 23.7g; Protein: 21.3g; Fat: 9.9g; Fiber: 8.8g

White Chicken Chili

Serves: 8
Preparation Time: 5 minutes
Cooking Time: 20 minutes

Ingredients
- 2 tablespoons oil
- 2 pounds chicken thighs
- 1 onion, diced
- 3 cloves of garlic, minced
- 1 cup chicken broth
- 2 cans northern beans, undrained
- 1 cup corn kernels
- 1 packet taco seasoning
- 1 can chopped green chilies
- 1 can condensed cream of chicken soup
- 1 cup Monterey Jack cheese, grated
- Salt and pepper to taste

Instructions
1. Press the Sauté button on the Instant Pot.
2. Stir in the chicken thighs, onions, and garlic until fragrant.
3. Add the rest of the ingredients.
4. Close the lid and press the Manual button.
5. Adjust the cooking time to 15 minutes.
6. Do natural pressure release.

Nutrition information:
Calories per serving: 608; Carbohydrates: 38.1g; Protein: 41.2g; Fat:32.4g; Fiber: 10.6g

Instant Pot Turkey Chili

Serves: 6
Preparation Time: 5 minutes
Cooking Time: 15 minutes

Ingredients
- 2 tablespoons olive oil
- 1-pound ground turkey
- 1 onion, diced
- 3 cloves of garlic, minced
- 3 stalks of celery, diced
- 1 green bell pepper, diced
- 3 carrots, peeled and sliced
- 1 can crushed tomatoes
- 1 can black beans, drained and rinsed
- 1 can chopped green chilies, drained
- ½ cup water
- 3 tablespoons chili powder
- 1 ½ teaspoon ground cumin
- Salt and pepper

Instructions
1. Press the Sauté button on the Instant Pot.
2. Heat the oil and stir in the ground turkey, onions, and garlic until fragrant.
3. Stir in the celery, bell pepper, carrots, and the rest of the ingredients.
4. Close the lid and press the Manual button.
5. Adjust the cooking time to 10 minutes.
6. Do natural pressure release.

Nutrition information:
Calories per serving: 453; Carbohydrates: 45.8g; Protein: 34.2g; Fat: 17.6g; Fiber: 16.1g

Cheesy Chili Mac

Serves: 8
Preparation Time: 5 minutes
Cooking Time: 15 minutes

Ingredients
- 1 tablespoon vegetable oil
- 1 onion, diced
- 3 cloves of garlic, minced
- 1-pound ground beef
- 1 red bell pepper, diced
- 1 jalapeno, diced
- 2 tablespoons chili powder
- ¼ teaspoon cayenne pepper
- 2 cups water
- 1 can diced tomatoes
- 8 ounces elbow macaroni
- 1 cup corn kernels
- 2 tablespoons cilantro, chopped
- Salt and pepper
- 1 ½ cups Monterey Jack cheese, grated

Instructions
1. Press the Sauté button on the Instant Pot.
2. Heat the oil and stir in the onions, garlic, and ground beef. Stir until well combined.
3. Add the rest of the ingredients and give a good stir.
4. Close the lid and press the Manual button.
5. Adjust the cooking time to 15 minutes.
6. Do natural pressure release.

Nutrition information:
Calories per serving: 392; Carbohydrates:29.3 g; Protein: 25.4g; Fat: 19.8g; Fiber: 3g

Seafood Recipes

Salmon and Veggies

Serves: 1
Preparation Time: 3 minutes
Cooking Time: 10 minutes

Ingredients
- 1 cup sliced vegetables
- 1 salmon fillet, about 7 ounces
- A dash of salmon seasoning
- ½ teaspoon chicken bullion
- ¼ cup dry sherry
- Salt and pepper

Instructions
1. Place the vegetables in a baking pan that will fit inside the Instant Pot.
2. Season the salmon fillets with salmon seasoning. Sprinkle with chicken bouillon.
3. Place the salmon on top of the vegetables.
4. Pour the sherry and season with salt and pepper to taste.
5. Place the baking dish inside the Instant Pot.
6. Pour a cup of water around the baking dish.
7. Close the lid and press the Steam button.
8. Adjust the cooking time to 10 minutes.
9. Do quick pressure release.

Nutrition information:
Calories per serving: 450; Carbohydrates: 42.5g; Protein: 41g; Fat: 12.6g; Fiber: 10.8g

Salmon and Rice Pilaf

Serves: 5
Preparation Time: 3 minutes
Cooking Time: 8 minutes

Ingredients
- ½ cup Jasmine rice
- ¼ cup dried vegetable soup mix
- 1 cup chicken broth
- 1 tablespoons salt
- 1 pinch saffron
- 12 6-ounce wild salmon fillets

Instructions
1. Place all ingredients in the Instant Pot.
2. Place a steamer rack above the rice and arrange the salmon fillets.
3. Season the salmon fillets with salt and pepper.
4. Close the lid and press the Rice button.
5. Adjust the cooking time to 8 minutes.
6. Do natural pressure release.

Nutrition information:
Calories per serving: 600; Carbohydrates: 7g; Protein: 79.8g; Fat: 27.4g; Fiber: 2.6g

Instant Pot Poached Salmon

Serves: 4
Preparation Time: 3 minutes
Cooking Time: 4minutes

Ingredients
- 16-ounce salmon fillet with skin
- 4 scallions, chopped
- Zest of 1 lemon
- ½ teaspoon fennel seeds
- 1 teaspoon white wine vinegar
- 1 bay leaf
- ½ cup dry white wine
- 2 cups chicken broth
- ¼ cup fresh dill
- Salt and pepper

Instructions
1. Place all ingredients in the Instant Pot.
2. Give a good stir.
3. Close the lid and press the Manual button.
4. Adjust the cooking time to 4 minutes.
5. Do natural pressure release.

Nutrition information:
Calories per serving:631; Carbohydrates: 3.6g; Protein: 98.2g; Fat: 24.3g; Fiber: 0.7g

Spicy Lemon Halibut

Serves: 4
Preparation Time: 5 minutes
Cooking Time: 8 minutes

Ingredients
- 4 halibut fillets
- 2 lemons, sliced
- 2 tablespoon chili pepper flakes
- Salt and pepper

Instructions
1. Place a trivet or steamer basket in the Instant Pot.
2. Pour a cup of water.
3. Season the halibut fillets with chili pepper flakes, salt, and pepper.
4. Place on the trivet and arrange slices of lemons.
5. Close the lid and press the Manual button.
6. Adjust the cooking time to 8 minutes.
7. Do natural pressure release.

Nutrition information:
Calories per serving: 770; Carbohydrates: 3.5g; Protein: 58.9g; Fat: 56.6g; Fiber: 0.4g

Instant Pot Salmon Fillet

Serves: 2
Preparation Time: 5 minutes
Cooking Time: 10 minutes
Ingredients
- 2 salmon fillets, skin on
- 2 teaspoon chipotles paste
- A handful of asparagus spears, trimmed
- 1 lemon, sliced

Instructions
1. Place a trivet or steamer basket in the Instant Pot.
2. Pour a cup of water.
3. Season the salmon fillets with chipotle paste.
4. Place on the steamer the asparagus and place the salmon fillets on top.
5. Arrange the lemon slices.
6. Close the lid and press the Steam button.
7. Adjust the cooking time to 10 minutes.
8. Do natural pressure release.

Nutrition information:
Calories per serving:400; Carbohydrates: 2.8g; Protein: 65.4g; Fat: 14.8g; Fiber: 0.3g

Simple Instant Pot Salmon

Serves: 2
Preparation Time: 3 minutes
Cooking Time: 10 minutes
Ingredients
- 2 salmon fillets
- Salt and pepper

Instructions
1. Place a trivet or steamer basket in the Instant Pot.
2. Pour a cup of water.
3. Season the salmon fillets with salt and pepper to taste.
4. Place on the steamer salmon fillets.
5. Close the lid and press the Steam button.
6. Adjust the cooking time to 10 minutes.
7. Do natural pressure release.

Nutrition information:
Calories per serving: 347; Carbohydrates: 0g; Protein: 46.8g; Fat: 16.3g; Fiber: 0g

Salmon with Lemon Caper Chimichurri

Serves: 4
Preparation Time: 30 minutes
Cooking Time: 15 minutes
Ingredients
- 2 tablespoons olive oil
- 1 teaspoon garlic, minced
- 2 anchovies
- ½ teaspoon crushed red pepper
- 1 tablespoon butter
- Juice and zest of 1 lemon
- 2 tablespoons capers
- 4 salmon fillets
- Salt and pepper to taste

Instructions
1. Place a trivet or steamer basket in the Instant Pot.
2. Pour a cup of water.
3. In a small bowl, combine all ingredients.
4. Marinate the salmon fillets for at least 30 minutes inside the fridge.
5. Once ready, place them on top of the steamer basket.
6. Close the lid and press the Steam button.
7. Adjust the cooking time to 15 minutes.
8. Do natural pressure release.

Nutrition information:
Calories per serving: 446; Carbohydrates: 2.4g; Protein: 47.8g; Fat: 26.8g; Fiber:0.4g

Asian Fish and Vegetables

Serves: 2
Preparation Time: 5 minutes
Cooking Time: 15 minutes
Ingredients
- ½ pound frozen vegetables of your choice
- 2 fillets of any white fish
- 1 clove of garlic, minced
- 2 teaspoons grated ginger
- ¼ long red chili, sliced
- 2 tablespoons soy sauce
- 1 tablespoon honey
- Salt and pepper

Instructions
1. Place a trivet or steamer basket in the Instant Pot.
2. Pour a cup of water.
3. Place the vegetables in a baking dish that will fit inside the Instant Pot.
4. Place the baking dish on top of the steamer basket.
5. For the fish, place the fish in a bowl and add the rest of the ingredients. Mix gently to combine.
6. Place the fish on top of the vegetables.
7. Close the lid and press the Steam button.
8. Adjust the cooking time to 15 minutes.
9. Do natural pressure release.

Nutrition information:
Calories per serving: 349; Carbohydrates: 30.5g; Protein: 25.7g; Fat: 13.9g; Fiber: 3.8g

Instant Pot Mediterranean Fish

Serves: 3
Preparation Time: 3 minutes
Cooking Time: 6 minutes
Ingredients
- ¼ cup red wine
- 1 tablespoon red wine vinegar
- 1 tablespoon lemon juice, freshly squeezed
- 1 clove of garlic, minced
- ¼ teaspoon dried oregano
- 1-pound salmon fillets, fresh
- 2 sprigs rosemary
- Salt and pepper
- 1 tablespoon feta cheese, crumbled

Instructions
1. Place all ingredients in the Instant Pot except for the feta cheese.
2. Close the lid and press the Manual button.
3. Adjust the cooking time to 6 minutes.
4. Do natural pressure release.
5. Once the lid is open, garnish with feta cheese on top.

Nutrition information:
Calories per serving: 377; Carbohydrates: 4.35g; Protein: 38.6g; Fat: 21.6g; Fiber: 0.4g

Thai Coconut Fish

Serves: 4
Preparation Time: 4 minutes
Cooking Time: 6 minutes
Ingredients
- 4 tilapia fillets, skin removed
- 1 cup coconut milk
- ½ teaspoon Thai green curry paste
- Tablespoon fish sauce
- Zest and juice of 1 lime
- 2 teaspoons brown sugar
- 1 teaspoon minced garlic
- 1 tablespoon fresh ginger, grated

Instructions
1. Place all ingredients in the Instant Pot.
2. Close the lid and press the Manual button.
3. Adjust the cooking time to 6 minutes.
4. Do natural pressure release.

Nutrition information:
Calories per serving:265; Carbohydrates: 7.3g; Protein: 25.1g; Fat: 16.3g; Fiber:1.6g

Fish with Orange and Ginger Sauce

Serves: 4
Preparation Time: 3 minutes
Cooking Time: 6 minutes
Ingredients
- 4 white fish fillets
- Juice and zest of 1 lemon
- 1 thumb-size ginger, grated
- 1 tablespoon olive oil
- Salt and pepper
- 1 cup fish stock
- 4 spring onions, chopped

Instructions
1. Place all ingredients except for the spring onions in the Instant Pot.
2. Close the lid and press the Manual button.
3. Adjust the cooking time to 6 minutes.
4. Do natural pressure release.
5. Once the lid is open, garnish the fish with spring onions.

Nutrition information:
Calories per serving: 235; Carbohydrates: 3.1g; Protein:22.5 g; Fat: 14.6g; Fiber:0.6 g

Fish Coconut Curry

Serves: 4
Preparation Time: 3 minutes
Cooking Time: 8 minutes
Ingredients
- 1 tablespoons olive oil
- ½ teaspoon mustard seeds
- 1-pound tilapia fillets, cut into thick strips
- 1 can coconut milk
- 1 tablespoon ginger, grated
- 15 curry leaves
- ½ onion, sliced
- ½ green pepper, sliced
- ½ yellow pepper, sliced
- ½ teaspoon turmeric powder
- 2 teaspoons coriander powder
- 1 teaspoon cumin powder
- 1 teaspoon garam masala
- Salt and pepper

Instructions
1. Press the Sauté button on the Instant Pot.
2. Heat the oil and fry the mustard seeds until they pop.
3. Pour in the rest of the ingredients.
4. Close the lid and press the Manual button.
5. Adjust the cooking time to 8 minutes.
6. Do natural pressure release.

Nutrition information:
Calories per serving: 296; Carbohydrates: 7.4g; Protein: 25g; Fat: 19.9g; Fiber: 2.1g

Green Chili Mahi Mahi

Serves: 2
Preparation Time: 3 minutes
Cooking Time: 8 minutes
Ingredients
- 2 Mahi Mahi fillets, fresh
- ¼ cup commercial enchilada sauce
- Salt and pepper
- 2 tablespoons butter

Instructions
1. Place all ingredients except for the butter in the Instant Pot.
2. Close the lid and press the Manual button.
3. Adjust the cooking time to 8 minutes.
4. Do quick pressure release.
5. Once the lid is open, add the butter.

Nutrition information:
Calories per serving: 368; Carbohydrates:11.1 g; Protein: 20.4g; Fat: 27.5g; Fiber: 6g

Wild Alaskan Cod

Serves: 4
Preparation Time: 3 minutes
Cooking Time: 8 minutes
Ingredients
- 1 large fillet wild Alaskan Cod
- 1 cup cherry tomatoes, chopped
- Salt and pepper to taste
- 2 tablespoons butter

Instructions
1. Place all ingredients except for the butter in the Instant Pot.
2. Close the lid and press the Manual button.
3. Adjust the cooking time to 8 minutes.
4. Do quick pressure release.
5. Once the lid is open, add the butter.

Nutrition information:
Calories per serving:135; Carbohydrates: 1.4g; Protein: 17.6g; Fat: 6.2g; Fiber: 0.2g

Old Bay Fish Tacos

Serves: 4
Preparation Time: 3 minutes
Cooking Time: 8 minutes
Ingredients
- 2 large cod fillets
- 1 tablespoon old bay seasoning
- 1/2 cup quesadilla cheese

Instructions

1. Place a trivet or a steamer basket in the Instant Pot. Pour a cup of water.
2. Season the cod fillets with old bay seasoning.
3. Place on top of the steamer rack.
4. Close the lid and press the Steam button.
5. Adjust the cooking time to 10 minutes.
6. Do quick pressure release.
7. Serve with quesadilla cheese on top.

Nutrition information:
Calories per serving:82; Carbohydrates: 4g; Protein: 10.5g; Fat: 2.4g; Fiber: 0.3g

Instant Pot Mok Pa

Serves: 3
Preparation Time: 10 minutes
Cooking Time: 15 minutes

Ingredients
- 3 tablespoon sticky rice, soaked in water
- 1 stalk lemongrass, sliced
- 1 small shallot, chopped
- 2 cloves of garlic, minced
- 5 Thai bird chilies
- 2 tablespoons water
- 12 kaffir lime leaves
- 2 tablespoons fish sauce
- 1 banana leaf, washed
- 2 pounds white fish fillet
- 1 tablespoon green onions
- 1 cup fresh dill leaves, chopped
- ½ cup cilantro leaves, chopped

Instructions
1. Place in a mortar or food processor the rice, lemongrass, shallots, garlic, birth chilies, water, kaffir lime leaves, and fish sauce. Pulse until fine. Set aside.
2. Lay down the banana leaves on a leveled surface and place fish in the middle. Pour the rice mixture on top and garnish with green onions, dill, and cilantro leaves.
3. Fold the banana leaf and secure with a string. You can even wrap aluminum foil over.
4. Place a steamer basket in the Instant Pot and pour water over.
5. Place the fish wrapped in banana leaf on the steamer rack.
6. Close the lid and press the Steam button.
7. Adjust the cooking time to 15 minutes.
8. Do quick pressure release.

Nutrition information:
Calories per serving: 552; Carbohydrates: 16.9g; Protein: 57.2g; Fat: 28.2g; Fiber: 1g

Chinese-Style Steamed Ginger Scallion Fish

Serves: 5
Preparation Time: 5 minutes
Cooking Time: 15 minutes

Ingredients
- 3 tablespoons soy sauce
- 2 tablespoons rice wine
- 1 tablespoon Chinese black bean paste
- 1 teaspoon minced ginger
- 1 teaspoon garlic
- 1-pound firm white fish

Instructions
1. Place a trivet or a steamer basket in the Instant Pot. Pour a cup of water.
2. Place all ingredients in a baking dish that will fit in the Instant Pot.
3. Make sure that the fish is coated with the marinade.
4. Place the baking dish on top of the steamer rack.
5. Close the lid and press the Steam button.
6. Adjust the cooking time to 15 minutes.
7. Do quick pressure release.

Nutrition information:
Calories per serving: 188; Carbohydrates: 4.4g; Protein: 17.9g; Fat: 10.9g; Fiber: 0.9g

Sweet and Spicy Mahi Mahi

Serves: 2
Preparation Time: 4 minutes
Cooking Time: 15 minutes

Ingredients
- 2 Mahi Mahi fillets
- Salt and pepper
- 2 cloves of garlic, minced
- 1 thumb-size ginger, grated
- ½ lime, juiced
- 2 tablespoons honey
- 1 tablespoon Nanami Togarashi
- 2 tablespoons sriracha
- 1 tablespoon orange juice, freshly squeezed

Instructions
1. Place a trivet or a steamer basket in the Instant Pot. Pour a cup of water.
2. Place all ingredients in a baking dish that will fit in the Instant Pot.
3. Make sure that the fish is coated with the marinade.
4. Place the baking dish on top of the steamer rack.
5. Close the lid and press the Steam button.
6. Adjust the cooking time to 15 minutes.
7. Do quick pressure release.

Nutrition information:
Calories per serving: 331; Carbohydrates:30 g; Protein: 20.4g; Fat: 15.4g; Fiber: 5.8g

Lemon and Dill Fish Packets

Serves: 2
Preparation Time: 5 minutes
Cooking Time: 15 minutes

Ingredients
- 2 tilapia fillets
- Salt and pepper
- 2 sprigs fresh dill
- 4 slices of lemon
- 2 tablespoons butter

Instructions
1. Lay a large parchment paper on a surface.
2. Place the fillet in the middle of the parchment paper.
3. Season with salt and pepper. Add fresh dill and lemon slices on top.
4. Place the butter.
5. Place a trivet or a steamer basket in the Instant Pot.
6. Close the lid and press the Steam button.
7. Adjust the cooking time to 15 minutes.
8. Do quick pressure release.

Nutrition information:
Calories per serving: 244; Carbohydrates: 8.9g; Protein: 24.1g; Fat: 13.8g; Fiber: 0.7g

Instant Pot Shrimps

Serves: 8
Preparation Time: 1 minute
Cooking Time: 3 minutes
Ingredients
- 2 pounds shrimp
- 2 tablespoons butter
- 1 tablespoon garlic, minced
- ½ cup white wine
- ½ cup chicken stock
- 1 tablespoon lemon juice
- Salt and pepper
- 1 tablespoon parsley for garnish

Instructions
1. Place all ingredients in the Instant Pot.
2. Close the lid and press the Manual button.
3. Adjust the cooking time to 3 minutes.
4. Do quick pressure release.

Nutrition information:
Calories per serving: 150; Carbohydrates: 1.8g; Protein: 23.5g; Fat: 4.6g; Fiber: 0.2g

Instant Pot Shrimp Boil

Serves: 10
Preparation Time: 3 minutes
Cooking Time: 6 minutes
Ingredients
- 6 corn on the cobs, halved
- 12 ounces sausages
- 1 cup chicken broth
- 1 tablespoon old bay seasoning
- 1 teaspoon crushed red peppers
- 1 onion, chopped
- 2-pound shrimps
- Salt and pepper

Instructions
1. Place the corn and sausages in the Instant Pot.
2. Pour the chicken broth, old bay seasoning, red peppers, onions, and shrimps. Season with salt and pepper to taste.
3. Close the lid and press the Manual button.
4. Adjust the cooking time to 6 minutes.
5. Do quick pressure release.

Nutrition information:
Calories per serving:260; Carbohydrates:13.9 g; Protein: 31.5g; Fat: 9.4g; Fiber: 2.3g

Instant Pot Jambalaya

Serves: 10
Preparation Time: 3 minutes
Cooking Time: 10 minutes
Ingredients
- 1-pound smoked sausages, sliced
- 1-pound medium-sized shrimps, peeled and deveined
- 1 onion, diced
- 3 stalks of celery, chopped
- 3 cloves of garlic, minced
- 1 can diced tomatoes, juice included
- 1 ¼ cup long grain white rice
- ¾ cup water
- 1 teaspoon Cajun seasoning
- ¼ teaspoon crushed red pepper
- Salt and pepper
- 2 scallions, chopped

Instructions
1. Place all ingredients in the Instant Pot except for the scallions.
2. Give a good stir to combine everything.
3. Close the lid and press the Manual button.
4. Adjust the cooking time to 10 minutes.
5. Do quick pressure release.

Nutrition information:
Calories per serving:247; Carbohydrates: 26.4g; Protein: 16.7g; Fat: 8.9g; Fiber: 1.5g

Shrimps in Lobsters Sauce

Serves: 8
Preparation Time: 2 minutes
Cooking Time: 3 minutes
Ingredients
- 1 ½ pounds large shrimps, peeled and deveined
- 1 ½ cups lobster broth
- ½ tablespoon soy sauce
- ½ tablespoon Shaoxing wine
- 1 teaspoon sugar
- ½ teaspoon white pepper
- ½ tablespoon crushed garlic
- 2 eggs, beaten
- ½ tablespoon heavy cream

Instructions
1. Place all ingredients in the Instant Pot.
2. Give a good stir.
3. Close the lid and press the Manual button.
4. Adjust the cooking time to 3 minutes.
5. Do quick pressure release.

Nutrition information:
Calories per serving: 124; Carbohydrates: 6.1g; Protein: 6.8g; Fat:7.5 g; Fiber: 0.9g

Crabs in Coconut Milk

Serves: 6
Preparation Time: 2 minutes
Cooking Time: 6 minutes
Ingredients
- 1-pound crabs halved
- 1 can coconut milk
- 1 lemongrass stalk
- 1 thumb-size ginger, sliced
- 1 onion, chopped
- 3 cloves of garlic, minced
- Salt and pepper

Instructions
1. Place all ingredients in the Instant Pot.
2. Close the lid and press the Manual button.
3. Adjust the cooking time to 6 minutes.
4. Do quick pressure release.

Nutrition information:
Calories per serving:171; Carbohydrates: 5.3g; Protein: 14.9g; Fat:10.4g; Fiber: 1.4g

Steamed Shrimps and Asparagus in Instant Pot

Serves: 6
Preparation Time: 5 minutes
Cooking Time: 10 minutes

Ingredients
- 1-pound shrimps, peeled and deveined
- 1 bunch asparagus, trimmed
- 1 teaspoon oil
- ½ tablespoon Cajun seasoning

Instructions
1. Place a trivet or a steamer basket in the Instant Pot. Pour a cup of water.
2. Place all ingredients in a baking dish that will fit in the Instant Pot.
3. Mix to combine everything.
4. Place the baking dish on the steamer basket.
5. Close the lid and press the Steam button.
6. Adjust the cooking time to 10 minutes.
7. Do quick pressure release.

Nutrition information:
Calories per serving: 89; Carbohydrates: 1.3g; Protein: 16g; Fat: 1.8g; Fiber: 0.6g

Instant Pot Seafood Stew

Serves: 6
Preparation Time: 5 minutes
Cooking Time: 10 minutes

Ingredients
- 3 tablespoons olive oil
- 1 onion, sliced
- 2 cloves of garlic, minced
- 1 ½ pounds cod, sliced into strips
- 1-pound shrimps, peeled and deveined
- 12 neck clams, cleaned
- 2 bay leaves
- 2 teaspoons paprika
- 1 green bell pepper, sliced
- 1 ½ cups tomatoes diced
- 1 cup fish stock
- Salt and pepper

Instructions
1. Press the Sauté button on the Instant Pot.
2. Heat the oil and sauté the onions and garlic until fragrant.
3. Add the fish, shrimps, and clams. Stir for a few minutes.
4. Pour in the rest of the ingredients.
5. Close the lid and press the Manual button.
6. Adjust the cooking time to 10 minutes.
7. Do quick pressure release.

Nutrition information:
Calories per serving: 262; Carbohydrates: 4.8g; Protein: 38.6g; Fat: 9.1g; Fiber: 1g

Japanese Seafood Curry

Serves: 4
Preparation Time: 5 minutes
Cooking Time: 18 minutes

Ingredients
- 3 onions, chopped
- 2 cloves of garlic, minced
- 1-inch ginger, grated
- 3 cups water
- 1 2-inch long kombu or dried kelp
- 6 shiitake mushrooms, halved
- 12 manila clams, scrubbed
- 6 ounces medium-sized shrimps, peeled and deveined
- 6 ounces bay scallops
- ¼ cup white wine
- 1 package Japanese curry roux
- ¼ apple, sliced

Instructions
1. Dump the onions, garlic, ginger, water, kombu, and mushrooms in the Instant Pot.
2. Close the lid and press the Manual button. Adjust the cooking time to 10 minutes to bring out the flavor of the stock.
3. Do quick pressure release.
4. Once the lid is open, remove the kombu and add the rest of the ingredients.
5. Give a good stir.
6. Close the lid and press the Manual button.
7. Adjust the cooking time to 8 minutes.
8. Do quick pressure release.

Nutrition information:
Calories per serving: 158; Carbohydrates: 17.5g; Protein: 20.1g; Fat: 1.2g; Fiber: 2.3g

Clams and Corn

Serves: 6
Preparation Time: 3 minutes
Cooking Time: 10 minutes

Ingredients
- 1-pound clams, scrubbed
- 2 corns on the cob, halved
- ½ cup dry white wine
- 4 cloves of garlic, minced
- 1 cup water

Instructions
1. Place all ingredients in the Instant Pot.
2. Close the lid and press the Manual button.
3. Adjust the cooking time to 10 minutes.
4. Do natural pressure release.

Nutrition information:
Calories per serving: 86; Carbohydrates: 14 g; Protein: 3.2g; Fat: 2.3g; Fiber: 0.9g

Steamed Crab Legs

Serves: 4
Preparation Time:
Cooking Time:

Ingredients
- 2 pounds frozen crab legs
- 4 tablespoons butter
- 1 tablespoon lemon juice, freshly squeezed

Instructions
1. Place a trivet or a steamer basket in the Instant Pot. Pour a cup of water.
2. Arrange the crab legs on it.
3. Close the lid and press the Steam button.
4. Adjust the cooking time to 4 minutes.
5. Do quick pressure release.
6. Once the lid is open, check if the crab legs are bright pink.

7. Serve crab legs with butter and a drizzle of lemon juice.
Nutrition information:
Calories per serving: 291; Carbohydrates: 0.3g; Protein: 41g; Fat: 12.3g; Fiber: 0g

Lobster with Wine and Tomatoes

Serves: 4
Preparation Time: 5 minutes
Cooking Time: 10 minutes
Ingredients
- 4 tablespoons olive oil
- 2 onions, diced
- 2 cloves of garlic, minced
- 1 carrot, chopped
- 2 lobsters, shelled
- ½ cup cognac
- 1-pound ripe tomatoes
- 2 tablespoon tomato paste
- 1/3 clam juice
- 1 tablespoon tarragon

Instructions
1. Press the Sauté button on the Instant Pot.
2. Heat the oil and sauté the onions and garlic until fragrant.
3. Add the rest of the ingredients.
4. Stir to combine.
5. Close the lid and press the Manual button.
6. Adjust the cooking time to 10 minutes.
7. Do quick pressure release.

Nutrition information:
Calories per serving: 300; Carbohydrates: 13.2g; Protein: 14.9g; Fat: 14.5g; Fiber: 3.1g

Instant Pot Mussels

Serves: 6
Preparation Time: 3 minutes
Cooking Time: 6 minutes
Ingredients
- 1 cup white wine
- 3 Roma tomatoes, chopped
- 2 cloves of garlic, minced
- 1 bay leaf
- 2 pounds mussels, scrubbed
- ½ cup fresh parsley, chopped
- Salt and pepper

Instructions
1. Place all ingredients in the Instant Pot.
2. Close the lid and press the Manual button.
3. Adjust the cooking time to 6 minutes.
4. Do natural pressure release.

Nutrition information:
Calories per serving: 155; Carbohydrates: 10.5g; Protein: 19.5g; Fat: 3.7g; Fiber: 1.1g

Instant Pot Boiled Octopus

Serves: 8
Preparation Time: 3 minutes
Cooking Time: 15 minutes
Ingredients
- 2 ½ pounds whole octopus, sliced and cleaned
- Salt and pepper to taste
- 3 tablespoons lemon juice, freshly squeezed
- 1 cup water

Instructions
1. Place all ingredients in the Instant Pot.
2. Close the lid and press the Manual button.
3. Adjust the cooking time to 15 minutes.
4. Do quick pressure release.

Nutrition information:
Calories per serving: 90; Carbohydrates: 7.7g; Protein: 4.6g; Fat: 6.1g; Fiber: 0.1g

Instant Pot Lobster Roll

Serves: 6
Preparation Time: 5 minutes
Cooking Time: 6 minutes
Ingredients
- 1 ½ cups chicken broth
- 1 teaspoon old bay seasoning
- 2 pounds lobster tails, raw and in the shell
- 1 lemon, halved
- 3 scallions, chopped
- ½ cup mayonnaise
- 4 tablespoons unsalted butter
- ¼ teaspoon celery salt

Instructions
1. Pour the broth into the Instant Pot and sprinkle with old bay seasoning.
2. Place a steamer on top and lay each lobster tail shell side down.
3. Squeeze the first half of the lemon over the lobsters.
4. Close the lid and press the Manual button.
5. Adjust the cooking time to 6 minutes.
6. While cooking, prepare the sauce by combining the rest of the ingredients in a bowl.
7. Once the timer beeps off, do quick pressure release.
8. Brush the mayo dip on the exposed meat of the lobster tails.

Nutrition information:
Calories per serving: 392; Carbohydrates: 2.7g; Protein: 47.5g; Fat: 20.2g; Fiber: 0.6g

Instant Pot Easy Scallops

Serves: 3
Preparation Time: 5 minutes
Cooking Time: 6 minutes
Ingredients
- 1 tablespoon oil
- 1-pound sea scallops, shells removed
- ½ cup coconut aminos
- 3 tablespoons maple syrup
- ½ teaspoon garlic powder
- ½ teaspoon ground ginger
- ½ teaspoon salt

Instructions
1. Place a trivet or a steamer basket in the Instant Pot. Pour a cup of water.
2. In a baking dish that will fit the Instant Pot, pour all the ingredients.
3. Place the baking dish on top of the steamer.
4. Close the lid and press the Steam button.
5. Adjust the cooking time to 6 minutes.
6. Do quick pressure release.

Nutrition information:

Calories per serving: 270; Carbohydrates: 2.1g; Protein: 25g; Fat:16g; Fiber: 0g

Instant Pot Tuna Casserole

Serves: 4
Preparation Time: 3 minutes
Cooking Time: 15 minutes
Ingredients
- 2 carrots, peeled and chopped
- ¼ cup diced onions
- 1 cup frozen peas
- ¾ cup milk
- 2 cans tuna, drained
- 1 can cream of celery soup
- 2 tablespoons butter
- ½ cup water
- 2 eggs beaten
- Salt and pepper

Instructions
1. Place all ingredients in the Instant Pot.
2. Stir to combine.
3. Close the lid and press the Manual button.
4. Adjust the cooking time to 15 minutes.
5. Do quick pressure release.

Nutrition information:
Calories per serving:305; Carbohydrates: 15.3g; Protein: 24.5g; Fat: 16.5g; Fiber: 2.8g

Lemon Shrimps with Veggies and Parmesan

Serves: 4
Preparation Time: 5 minutes
Cooking Time: 3 minutes
Ingredients
- 1 tablespoons butter
- ½ cup onion, chopped
- 3 cloves of garlic, minced
- 1 pound's shrimps, peeled and deveined
- ½ cup parmesan cheese
- 1 cup spinach, shredded
- ½ cup chicken broth
- ½ cup dry white wine
- Salt and pepper

Instructions
1. Press the Sauté button on the Instant Pot.
2. Heat the oil and sauté the onion and garlic until fragrant.
3. Stir in the rest of the ingredients.
4. Give a good stir.
5. Close the lid and press the Manual button.
6. Adjust the cooking time to 3 minutes.
7. Do quick pressure release.

Nutrition information:
Calories per serving: 294; Carbohydrates: 5.6g; Protein: 36.8g; Fat: 13.2g; Fiber: 0.7g

Mediterranean-Style Cod

Serves: 6
Preparation Time: 3 minutes
Cooking Time: 10 minutes
Ingredients
- 3 tablespoons butter
- 1 onion, sliced
- 1 ½ pounds fresh cod fillets
- Salt and pepper
- 1 lemon juice, freshly squeezed
- 1 can diced tomatoes

Instructions
1. Press the Sauté button on the Instant Pot.
2. Heat the oil and sauté the onion until fragrant.
3. Stir in the rest of the ingredients.
4. Give a good stir.
5. Close the lid and press the Manual button.
6. Adjust the cooking time to 10 minutes.
7. Do natural pressure release.

Nutrition information:
Calories per serving: 140; Carbohydrates: 2.5g; Protein:17.8g; Fat: 6.4g; Fiber:0.8g

Coconut Curry Sea Bass

Serves: 3
Preparation Time: 3 minutes
Cooking Time: 10 minutes
Ingredients
- 1 can coconut milk
- Juice of 1 lime, freshly squeezed
- 1 tablespoon red curry paste
- 1 teaspoon fish sauce
- 1 teaspoon coconut aminos
- 1 teaspoon honey
- 2 teaspoons sriracha
- 2 cloves of garlic, minced
- 1 teaspoon ground turmeric
- 1 tablespoon curry powder
- ¼ cup fresh cilantro
- Salt and pepper

Instructions
1. Put all ingredients in the Instant Pot.
2. Give a good stir.
3. Close the lid and press the Manual button.
4. Adjust the cooking time to 10 minutes.
5. Do natural pressure release.

Nutrition information:
Calories per serving: 222; Carbohydrates: 12.9g; Protein: 3.1g; Fat: 18.7g; Fiber: 4.7g

Creamy Haddock with Kale

Serves: 5
Preparation Time: 4 minutes
Cooking Time: 10 minutes
Ingredients
- 2 tablespoons butter
- 1 onion, chopped
- 2 cloves of garlic, minced
- 2 cups chicken broth
- 1 teaspoon crushed red pepper flakes
- 1-pound wild Haddock fillets
- ½ cup heavy cream
- 1 tablespoons basil
- 1 cup kale leaves, chopped
- Salt and pepper to taste

Instructions
1. Press the Sauté button on the Instant Pot.
2. Heat the butter and sauté the onion until fragrant.
3. Stir in the rest of the ingredients.
4. Give a good stir.

5. Close the lid and press the Manual button.
6. Adjust the cooking time to 10 minutes.
7. Do quick pressure release.
Nutrition information:
Calories per serving: 327; Carbohydrates: 5.5g; Protein: 36.8 g; Fat: 16.2g; Fiber: 2.4g

Steamed Fish Patra Ni Maachi

Serves: 4
Preparation Time: 3 minutes
Cooking Time: 10 minutes
Ingredients
- 1-pound tilapia fillets
- ½ cup green commercial chutney

Instructions
1. Place a trivet or a steamer basket in the Instant Pot. Pour a cup of water.
2. Cut a large parchment paper and place the fish in the middle.
3. Pour over the green chutney.
4. Fold and secure the parchment paper.
5. Place on top of the steamer basket.
6. Close the lid and press the Manual button.
7. Adjust the cooking time to 10 minutes.
8. Do natural pressure release.
Nutrition information:
Calories per serving: 134; Carbohydrates: 11g; Protein: 22g; Fat: 3g; Fiber: 0g

Beef Recipes

Asian Pot Roast

Serves: 6
Preparation Time: 5 minutes
Cooking Time: 60 minutes
Ingredients
- 3 pounds chuck roast, trimmed from fat
- 2 tablespoons olive oil
- 3 cloves of garlic
- 1 onion, diced
- 2 tablespoons ginger, minced
- ¼ cup soy sauce
- 2 tablespoons honey
- 2/3 cup water
- ¼ cup cilantro, chopped

Instructions
1. Press the Sauté button on the Instant Pot.
2. Heat the oil and sauté the garlic, onions, and ginger until fragrant.
3. Add in the chuck roast and sear for at least 3 minutes on all sides.
4. Pour in the soy sauce honey, and water.
5. Close the lid and press the Meat/Stew button.
6. Adjust the cooking time to 60 minutes.
7. Do natural pressure release.
8. Open the lid and garnish with cilantro on top.
Nutrition information:
Calories per serving: 518; Carbohydrates: 11g; Protein: 61.6g; Fat: 26.8g; Fiber: 0.6g

Italian Pot Roast

Serves: 8
Preparation Time: 5 minutes
Cooking Time: 60 minutes
Ingredients
- 8 ounces bacon, diced
- 2 onions, chopped
- 6 cloves of garlic, minced
- 2 teaspoons dried oregano
- 1 teaspoon tomato paste
- 1 package cremini mushrooms, sliced
- ½ cup dried red wine
- 1 can crushed tomatoes
- 1 cup chicken broth
- 2 bay leaves
- 2 pounds boneless beef chuck roast
- Salt and pepper to taste

Instructions
1. Press the Sauté button on the Instant Pot and add the bacon. Cook the bacon until it has rendered its fat. Set the bacon aside.
2. Use the bacon fat and sauté the onions and garlic until fragrant.
3. Add the oregano, tomato paste, mushrooms, and the rest of the ingredients.
4. Close the lid and press the Meat/Stew button.
5. Adjust the cooking time to 60 minutes.
6. Do natural pressure release.
7. Open the lid and garnish with parsley if desired.
Nutrition information:
Calories per serving: 380; Carbohydrates: 11.1g; Protein: 40.7g; Fat: 20.1g; Fiber: 2.5g

Simple Instant Pot Roast

Serves: 8
Preparation Time: 5 minutes
Cooking Time: 1 hour and 15 minutes
Ingredients
- 2 tablespoons oil
- 3 cloves of garlic, minced
- 1 onion, chopped
- 3 pounds chuck roast
- 1/3 cup tomato paste
- 2 carrots, chopped
- 2 stalks of celery, chopped
- 2 sprigs of thyme
- 2 bay leaves
- 2 cups beef stock
- ¼ cup dried porcini mushrooms, rehydrated
- ½ cup boiling water
- 1 tablespoon red wine vinegar
- Salt and pepper

Instructions
1. Press the Sauté button on the Instant Pot and heat the oil.
2. Sauté the garlic and onions until fragrant.
3. Add in the chuck roast and sear until all sides turn gold in color.
4. Add the rest of the ingredients and season with salt and pepper to taste.
5. Close the lid and press the Meat/Stew button.
6. Adjust the cooking time to 60 minutes.
7. Do natural pressure release.
Nutrition information:
Calories per serving: 385; Carbohydrates: 8.4g; Protein: 47.9g; Fat: 19.2g; Fiber: 1.6g

Classic Pot Roast

Serves: 4
Preparation Time: 5 minutes
Cooking Time: 1 hour and 15 minutes
Ingredients
- 2 tablespoons unsalted butter
- 2 medium onions, sliced
- 4 cloves of garlic, crushed
- 1 boneless chuck eye roast
- 1 cup baby carrots, peeled
- 1 stalk of celery, chopped
- 1 cup beef broth
- ½ cup red wine
- 1 tablespoon tomato paste
- 1 bay leaf
- 1 tablespoon balsamic vinegar
- Salt and pepper

Instructions
1. Press the Sauté button on the Instant Pot and heat the butter.
2. Sauté the garlic and onions until fragrant.
3. Add in the chuck eye roast and sear all sides.
4. Stir in the rest of the ingredients.
5. Close the lid and press the Meat/Stew button.
6. Adjust the cooking time to 60 minutes.
7. Do natural pressure release.

Nutrition information:
Calories per serving: 361; Carbohydrates: 9.6g; Protein: 41.8g; Fat: 16.8g; Fiber: 0.7g

Sunday Pot Roast

Serves: 9
Preparation Time: 5 minutes
Cooking Time: 1 hour and 15 minutes
Ingredients
- 4 tablespoons olive oil
- 1 onion, quartered
- 3 pounds beef chuck roast
- 1 package onion soup mix
- 2 cups beef broth
- 1-pound baby potatoes, scrubbed
- Salt and pepper

Instructions
1. Press the Sauté button on the Instant Pot and heat the oil.
2. Sauté the onions until fragrant.
3. Add in the chuck roast and sear all sides.
4. Stir in the rest of the ingredients.
5. Close the lid and press the Meat/Stew button.
6. Adjust the cooking time to 60 minutes.
7. Do natural pressure release.

Nutrition information:
Calories per serving: 396; Carbohydrates: 15.1g; Protein: 41.8g; Fat: 18.9g; Fiber:1.5 g

Balsamic Pot Roast

Serves: 10
Preparation Time: 5 minutes
Cooking Time: 1 hour and 15 minutes
Ingredients
- 4 pounds chuck roast
- Salt and pepper
- 1 tablespoon olive oil
- 2 onions, chopped
- 8 cloves of garlic, minced
- 1-pound baby potatoes, scrubbed
- 4 carrots, chopped
- 2 stalks of celery, chopped
- 1 cup beef broth
- ¼ cup balsamic vinegar
- 2 tablespoons Dijon mustard
- 1 tablespoon brown sugar
- 1 teaspoon bouillon powder

Instructions
1. Season the pot roast with salt and pepper.
2. Press the Sauté button on the Instant Pot and heat the oil.
3. Add the pot roast and sear all sides.
4. Stir in the onions and garlic until fragrant.
5. Add the rest of the ingredients.
6. Close the lid and press the Meat/Stew button.
7. Adjust the cooking time to 60 minutes.
8. Do natural pressure release.

Nutrition information:
Calories per serving:398; Carbohydrates: 14g; Protein:36 g; Fat: 21g; Fiber: 2g

Instant Pot Beef Mechado

Serves: 9
Preparation Time: 5 minutes
Cooking Time: 45 minutes
Ingredients
- 2 tablespoons oil
- 8 cloves of garlic, minced
- 1 large onion, chopped
- 3 pounds chuck roast, cut into chunks
- Salt and pepper
- 1 ½ cups beef broth
- ¼ cup soy sauce
- 1 bay leaf
- 4 medium potatoes, peeled and quartered
- ½ cup tomato sauce
- 1 cup ketchup

Instructions
1. Press the Sauté button on the Instant Pot.
2. Heat the oil and sauté the garlic and onions until fragrant.
3. Add in the chuck roast and stir to sear all edges.
4. Season with salt and pepper to taste.
5. Pour in the rest of the ingredients.
6. Close the lid and press the Meat/Stew button.
7. Adjust the cooking time to 40 minutes.
8. Do natural pressure release.

Nutrition information:
Calories per serving: 521; Carbohydrates: 47.1g; Protein: 45.4g; Fat: 17.4g; Fiber: 5.2g

Greek Style Beef Stew

Serves: 9
Preparation Time: 5 minutes
Cooking Time: 45 minutes
Ingredients
- 3 pounds beef shoulder, cut into chunks
- Salt and pepper
- ½ teaspoon marjoram
- 1 tablespoon dried basil

- 1 tablespoon oregano
- 1 teaspoon dill
- 1 onion, sliced
- 5 cloves of garlic, minced
- 1 cup beef broth
- ½ cup sun-dried tomatoes
- 1 teaspoon red wine vinegar
- ½ cup feta cheese, crumbled

Instructions
1. Place all ingredients in the Instant Pot except for the feta cheese.
2. Close the lid and press the Meat/Stew button.
3. Adjust the cooking time to 45 minutes.
4. Do natural pressure release.
5. Once the lid is open, garnish with feta cheese on top.

Nutrition information:
Calories per serving: 232; Carbohydrates: 5.6g; Protein: 34.7g; Fat: 8.4g; Fiber: 0.6g

Mississippi Coke Beef

Serves: 9
Preparation Time: 5 minutes
Cooking Time: 45 minutes

Ingredients
- 2 tablespoons oil
- 1 onion, chopped
- 5 cloves of garlic, minced
- 3 pounds beef stew meat, cut into chunks
- Salt and pepper
- 1 packet ranch dressing powder
- ½ cup beef broth
- 1 cup cola (your favorite brand)
- 1 tablespoon cornstarch + 2 tablespoons water

Instructions
1. Press the Sauté button on the Instant Pot.
2. Heat the oil and sauté the garlic and onions until fragrant.
3. Add the beef stew meat and sear all sides until lightly brown. Season with salt and pepper to taste.
4. Stir in the ranch dressing, broth, and cola.
5. Close the lid and press the Meat/Stew button.
6. Adjust the cooking time to 45 minutes.
7. Do natural pressure release.
8. Once the lid is open, press the Sauté button and add in the cornstarch slurry.
9. Allow simmering until the sauce thickens.

Nutrition information:
Calories per serving: 179; Carbohydrates: 9.6g; Protein: 0.9g; Fat: 15.8g; Fiber: 1g

Instant Pot Cheese Steak

Serves: 8
Preparation Time: 5 minutes
Cooking Time: 45 minutes

Ingredients
- 1 tablespoon oil
- 2 onions, sliced
- 3 pounds beef chuck roast, cut into chunks
- 2 green pepper, sliced
- 2 tablespoons steak seasoning
- 8 ounces mushrooms, sliced
- 1 cup beef stock
- Salt and pepper
- 1 cup mozzarella cheese

Instructions
1. Press the Sauté button on the Instant Pot.
2. Heat the oil and sauté the onions and beef chunks. Stir until the beef has seared on all sides.
3. Add the green peppers, steak seasoning, mushrooms, and beef stock.
4. Season with salt and pepper to taste.
5. Stir until well combined.
6. Add in mozzarella cheese on top.
7. Close the lid and press the Meat/Stew button.
8. Adjust the cooking time to 45 minutes.
9. Do natural pressure release.

Nutrition information:
Calories per serving: 425; Carbohydrates: 5g; Protein: 46.1g; Fat: 25.7g; Fiber: 1.5g

Instant Pot Sauerbraten (German-Style Beef)

Serves: 9
Preparation Time: 5 minutes
Cooking Time: 45 minutes

Ingredients
- 2 cups water
- 1 cup cider vinegar
- 1 cup red wine vinegar
- 1 onion, chopped
- 1 carrot, chopped
- 2 bay leaves
- 6 whole cloves
- ½ teaspoon ground mustard
- 3 pounds beef chuck roast, cut into chunks
- 1/3 cup sugar

Instructions
1. Place all ingredients in the Instant Pot except for the feta cheese.
2. Close the lid and press the Meat/Stew button.
3. Adjust the cooking time to 45 minutes.
4. Do natural pressure release.

Nutrition information:
Calories per serving: 310; Carbohydrates: 5.8g; Protein: 40.6g; Fat: 12.9g; Fiber: 0.4g

Chunky and Beanless Beef Chili

Serves: 6
Preparation Time:
Cooking Time: 1 hour and 15 minutes

Ingredients
- 1 tablespoon oil
- 2 pounds beef chuck roast, cut into cubes
- Salt and pepper
- 1 tablespoon chili powder
- 2 tablespoons cumin powder
- 1 tablespoon paprika
- 1 cup beef broth
- 8 ounces Portobello mushrooms, chopped
- 1 tablespoon onion powder
- 1 can tomato paste
- 1 can crushed tomatoes

Instructions
1. Press the Sauté button on the Instant Pot.

2. Heat the oil and sauté the beef chuck roast until lightly golden on all sides.
3. Season with salt and pepper to taste.
4. Stir in the rest of the ingredients.
5. Close the lid and press the Meat/Stew button.
6. Adjust the cooking time to 60 minutes.
7. Do natural pressure release.
Nutrition information:
Calories per serving:373; Carbohydrates: 15.4g; Protein: 44.8g; Fat:15.8 g; Fiber: 4g

BBQ Beef Ribs

Serves: 7
Preparation Time: 5 minutes
Cooking Time: 60 minutes
Ingredients
- 3 pounds beef ribs
- Salt and pepper
- 2 cups BBQ sauce
- 2 tablespoons pepper jelly
- ½ cup beef broth

Instructions
1. Season the ribs with salt and pepper.
2. Place in the Instant Pot and pour over the rest of the ingredients.
3. Close the lid and press the Meat/Stew button.
4. Adjust the cooking time to 60 minutes.
5. Do natural pressure release.
Nutrition information:
Calories per serving: 689; Carbohydrates: 10.1g; Protein: 32.2g; Fat: 58.3g; Fiber: 1.7g

Mocha-Rubbed Roast

Serves: 4
Preparation Time: 30 minutes
Cooking Time: 45 minutes
Ingredients
- 2 tablespoons ground coffee
- 2 tablespoons smoked paprika
- 1 tablespoon black pepper
- 1 teaspoon salt
- 1 tablespoon cocoa powder
- 1 teaspoon chili powder
- 1 teaspoon ground ginger
- 2 pounds beef chuck roast cut into cubes
- 1 cup beef broth
- 1 onion, chopped
- 6 dried figs, chopped
- 2 tablespoons balsamic vinegar

Instructions
1. In a mixing bowl, combine the first 7 ingredients.
2. Rub this spice mixture all over the beef and allow to marinate in the fridge for 30 minutes.
3. Place the marinated beef in the Instant Pot and pour in the rest of the ingredients.
4. Close the lid and press the Meat/Stew button.
5. Adjust the cooking time to 45 minutes.
6. Do natural pressure release.
Nutrition information:
Calories per serving: 408; Carbohydrates: 21.6g; Protein: 49.1g; Fat: 15.4g; Fiber: 4.1g

Poor Man's Pot Roast

Serves: 8
Preparation Time: 5 minutes
Cooking Time: 1 hour and 15 minutes
Ingredients
- 1 tablespoon olive oil
- 1 onion, chopped
- 3 cloves of garlic
- 3-pound beef pot roast
- 1 bag frozen vegetables of your choice
- 1 cup beef broth
- Salt and pepper

Instructions
1. Press the Sauté button on the Instant Pot.
2. Heat the oil and sauté the onions and garlic.
3. Stir in the beef pot roast and sear all sides until lightly golden.
4. Stir in the rest of the ingredients.
5. Close the lid and press the Meat/Stew button.
6. Adjust the cooking time to 60 minutes.
7. Do natural pressure release.
Nutrition information:
Calories per serving:282; Carbohydrates: 5.4g; Protein: 36.7g; Fat: 12.8g; Fiber: 0.9g

Italian Short Ribs

Serves: 8
Preparation Time: 5 minutes
Cooking Time: 60 minutes
Ingredients
- 2 tablespoons olive oil
- 1 ½ cups leeks, chopped
- 3 pounds short-ribs, bone in
- 1 teaspoon Italian seasoning
- Salt and pepper
- ½ cup dry white wine
- 1 ¼ cups pasta sauce

Instructions
1. Press the Sauté button on the Instant Pot.
2. Heat the olive oil and sauté the leeks.
3. Add in the short ribs and the rest of the ingredients.
4. Close the lid and press the Meat/Stew button.
5. Adjust the cooking time to 60 minutes.
6. Do natural pressure release.
Nutrition information:
Calories per serving: 341; Carbohydrates: 33.3g; Protein: 17.9g; Fat: 15.1g; Fiber: 3.7g

Korean Short Ribs

Serves: 10
Preparation Time: 5 minutes
Cooking Time: 45 minutes
Ingredients
- 5 pounds short ribs
- ½ cup coconut aminos
- 1 tablespoon rice vinegar
- 2 teaspoons fish sauce
- 1 medium pear, peeled and grated
- 6 cloves of garlic, minced
- 1 onion, chopped

- 1 thumb-size ginger, grated

Instructions
1. Place all ingredients in the Instant Pot except for the feta cheese.
2. Close the lid and press the Meat/Stew button.
3. Adjust the cooking time to 45 minutes.
4. Do natural pressure release.

Nutrition information:
Calories per serving: 363; Carbohydrates: 40.6g; Protein: 21.1g; Fat: 12.9g; Fiber: 4.3g

Basic Braised Beef Short Ribs

Serves: 12
Preparation Time: 5 minutes
Cooking Time: 45 minutes

Ingredients
- 1 tablespoon oil
- 1 onion, chopped
- 3 cloves of garlic, minced
- 4 pounds beef short ribs
- Salt and pepper to taste
- 1 cup water

Instructions
1. Press the Sauté button on the Instant Pot.
2. Heat the olive oil and sauté the onions.
3. Add in the short ribs and the rest of the ingredients.
4. Close the lid and press the Meat/Stew button.
5. Adjust the cooking time to 40 minutes.
6. Do natural pressure release.

Nutrition information:
Calories per serving: 260; Carbohydrates: 1.5g; Protein: 30.6g; Fat: 14.7g; Fiber: 0.2g

Asian Short Ribs

Serves: 12
Preparation Time: 5 minutes
Cooking Time: 45 minutes

Ingredients
- 2 tablespoons oil
- 12 short ribs
- ½ cup soy sauce
- ¼ cup ginger root, diced
- 6 ounces tomato paste
- 4 cloves of garlic, crushed
- ¼ cup raw honey
- 2 tablespoons sriracha

Instructions
1. Press the Sauté button on the Instant Pot.
2. Heat the oil and sauté the short ribs for 5 minutes.
3. Add the rest of the ingredients.
4. Close the lid and press the Meat/Stew button.
5. Adjust the cooking time to 40 minutes.
6. Do natural pressure release.

Nutrition information:
Calories per serving: 301; Carbohydrates: 3.5g; Protein: 28.3g; Fat: 19.2g; Fiber: 0.2g

Simple Bone-In Ribs

Serves: 4
Preparation Time: 5 minutes
Cooking Time: 45 minutes

Ingredients
- 4 large beef short ribs
- 1 onion, chopped
- 3 cloves of garlic, minced
- ½ cup apple juice
- 1 cup beef broth
- 2 tablespoons tomato paste
- Salt and pepper
- 1 tablespoon cornstarch + 2 tablespoons water

Instructions
1. Place all ingredients except for the cornstarch slurry in the Instant Pot.
2. Close the lid and press the Meat/Stew button.
3. Adjust the cooking time to 40 minutes.
4. Do natural pressure release.
5. Once the lid is open, press the Sauté button.
6. Stir in the cornstarch slurry and allow to simmer until the sauce thickens.

Nutrition information:
Calories per serving: 459; Carbohydrates: 15.3g; Protein: 45.2g; Fat: 24.8g; Fiber: 1.2g

Irish Beef Stew

Serves: 4
Preparation Time: 3 minutes
Cooking Time: 45 minutes

Ingredients
- 1-pound beef stew meat
- 1 ½ carrots, chopped
- 1 onion, chopped
- 4 cloves of garlic, minced
- 4 potatoes, diced
- 3 tablespoons paprika
- Salt and pepper
- 1 cup Guinness beer
- 1 cup beef broth

Instructions
1. Place all ingredients in the Instant Pot.
2. Close the lid and press the Meat/Stew button.
3. Adjust the cooking time to 45 minutes.
4. Do natural pressure release.

Nutrition information:
Calories per serving: 466; Carbohydrates: 82.2g; Protein: 10.6g; Fat: 9.2g; Fiber: 11.7g

Instant Pot Beef Burgundy

Serves: 12
Preparation Time: 5 minutes
Cooking Time: 45 minutes

Ingredients
- 5 slices of bacon
- 6-pound eye of round beef roast, cut into cubes
- 1 tablespoon olive oil
- 1 onion, chopped
- 1 cup mushrooms, sliced
- 1 carrot, chopped
- 5 cloves of garlic, minced
- 2 cups dry red wine
- ¾ cup beef stock

- ¼ cup soy sauce
- 2 teaspoons sugar
- 1 tablespoon thyme
- 2 tablespoons unsalted butter
- 2 bay leaves

Instructions
1. Place all ingredients in the Instant Pot.
2. Close the lid and press the Meat/Stew button.
3. Adjust the cooking time to 45 minutes.
4. Do natural pressure release.

Nutrition information:
Calories per serving: 515; Carbohydrates: 3.9g; Protein: 62.8g; Fat: 26.8g; Fiber: 0.5g

Sweet and Smoky Short Ribs

Serves: 6
Preparation Time: 5 minutes
Cooking Time: 50 minutes

Ingredients
- 2 tablespoons olive oil
- 1 onion, chopped
- 3 cloves of garlic, minced
- 3 pounds short ribs
- Salt and pepper
- 1 can rich stout beer
- 1/3 cup brown sugar
- 2 tablespoons tomato paste

Instructions
1. Press the Sauté button on the Instant Pot.
2. Heat the oil and sauté the onion and garlic.
3. Place the rest of the ingredients in the Instant Pot.
4. Close the lid and press the Meat/Stew button.
5. Adjust the cooking time to 45 minutes.
6. Do natural pressure release.

Nutrition information:
Calories per serving: 471; Carbohydrates: 53.7g; Protein: 21.6g; Fat: 17.8g; Fiber: 4.1g

Mexican Short Ribs

Serves: 8
Preparation Time: 3 minutes
Cooking Time: 45 minutes

Ingredients
- 1 teaspoon vegetable oil
- 1 onion, chopped
- 3 cloves of garlic, minced
- 4 pounds beef short ribs
- Salt and pepper
- 2 jalapeno peppers, chopped
- 1 tablespoon tomato paste
- 1 cup chicken stock
- 1 cup beer
- 1 can crushed tomatoes

Instructions
1. Press the Sauté button on the Instant Pot.
2. Heat the oil and sauté the onion and garlic.
3. Stir in the beef short ribs and sauté for another 3 minutes.
4. Place the rest of the ingredients in the Instant Pot.
5. Close the lid and press the Meat/Stew button.
6. Adjust the cooking time to 40 minutes.
7. Do natural pressure release.

Nutrition information:
Calories per serving: 456; Carbohydrates: 6.6g; Protein: 49.1g; Fat: 26.1g; Fiber: 1.1g

Korean Style Galbijjm

Serves: 6
Preparation Time: 5 minutes
Cooking Time: 45 minutes

Ingredients
- 2 pounds beef short ribs
- 1 tablespoon gochujang paste
- 3 tablespoons soy sauce
- 1 tablespoon brown sugar
- 3 cloves of garlic
- 1 tablespoon sesame oil
- 1 tablespoon mirin
- Salt and pepper

Instructions
1. Place all ingredients in the Instant Pot.
2. Close the lid and press the Meat/Stew button.
3. Adjust the cooking time to 45 minutes.
4. Do natural pressure release.

Nutrition information:
Calories per serving:385; Carbohydrates:4 g; Protein: 13g; Fat: 34g; Fiber: 0.8g

Vietnamese Beef Bo Kho

Serves: 4
Preparation Time: 3 minutes
Cooking Time: 45 minutes

Ingredients
- 1 onion, chopped
- 1-pound beef chuck stew meat, cut into chunks
- 2 tablespoons tomato paste
- 2 whole star anise
- 1 lemongrass stalk
- 1 tablespoon ginger, grated
- 1 tablespoon garlic, minced
- 1 ½ cups water
- ½ cups coconut water
- ½ teaspoon curry powder

Instructions
1. Place all ingredients in the Instant Pot.
2. Close the lid and press the Meat/Stew button.
3. Adjust the cooking time to 45 minutes.
4. Do natural pressure release.

Nutrition information:
Calories per serving:175; Carbohydrates: 8g; Protein: 15g; Fat: 9g; Fiber:2 g

Vegetable Beef Stew

Serves: 8
Preparation Time: 4 minutes
Cooking Time: 35 minutes

Ingredients
- 2 tablespoons oil
- 1 onion, diced
- 2 cloves of garlic

- 2 ½ pounds beef stew meat, cut into strips
- 2 carrots, sliced
- 3 potatoes, diced
- 1 cup green peas
- 1 cup corn kernels
- 1 can tomato sauce
- 1 bay leaf
- 2 tablespoons Worcestershire sauce
- Salt and pepper

Instructions
1. Press the Sauté button on the Instant Pot.
2. Heat the oil and sauté the onion and garlic.
3. Add in the beef stew meat and stir for another 3 minutes until lightly brown.
4. Close the lid and press the Meat/Stew button.
5. Adjust the cooking time to 30 minutes.
6. Do natural pressure release.

Nutrition information:
Calories per serving: 295; Carbohydrates: 34.8g; Protein: 4.8g; Fat: 15.9g; Fiber: 5.5g

Five Spice Beef Stew

Serves: 8
Preparation Time: 4 minutes
Cooking Time: 45 minutes

Ingredients
- 2 tablespoons oil
- 1 onion, diced
- 2 cloves of garlic, minced
- 2 pounds beef stew meat, cut into chunks
- Salt and pepper
- 1 tablespoon Chinese five spice powder
- 3 ½ cups beef broth
- 1 tablespoon cornstarch + 2 tablespoons water
- 1 tablespoon sesame seeds

Instructions
1. Press the Sauté button on the Instant Pot.
2. Heat the oil and sauté the onion and garlic.
3. Add in the beef stew meat and stir for another 3 minutes until lightly brown.
4. Season with salt and pepper to taste.
5. Add the five spice powder and beef broth.
6. Close the lid and press the Meat/Stew button.
7. Adjust the cooking time to 40 minutes.
8. Do natural pressure release.
9. Once the lid is open, press the Sauté button.
10. Stir in the cornstarch slurry and allow to simmer to thicken the sauce.
11. Garnish with sesame seeds.

Nutrition information:
Calories per serving:178; Carbohydrates: 13.1g; Protein:13.5g; Fat:5.8g; Fiber: 1.1g

Mole Beef Stew

Serves: 4
Preparation Time: 5 minutes
Cooking Time: 45 minutes

Ingredients
- 1 tablespoon olive oil
- 1 onion, chopped
- 3 cloves garlic, chopped
- 1 stalk celery, chopped
- 1 can plum tomatoes
- 1 cup vegetable stock
- ½ cup red wine
- 1-pound beef stew meat, cut into chunks
- 1 cup carrots, chopped
- ½ cup chocolate powder
- Salt and pepper

Instructions
1. Press the Sauté button on the Instant Pot.
2. Heat the oil and sauté the onion and garlic.
3. Add in the beef stew meat and stir for another 3 minutes until lightly brown.
4. Stir in the rest of the ingredients. Mix well to combine.
5. Close the lid and press the Meat/Stew button.
6. Adjust the cooking time to 40 minutes.
7. Do natural pressure release.

Nutrition information:
Calories per serving: 668; Carbohydrates: 15.6g; Protein:38.2g; Fat:15.8 g; Fiber: 2.4g

Instant Pot Carne Guisada

Serves: 4
Preparation Time: 5 minutes
Cooking Time: 45 minutes

Ingredients
- 2 tablespoons olive oil
- 1 onion, diced
- 1 tablespoon minced garlic
- 1-pound beef stew meat
- 1 serrano peppers, minced
- 1 bay leaf
- 1 ground cumin
- 1 teaspoon chili powder
- 1 teaspoon paprika
- Salt and pepper
- 1 cup beef stock
- ½ cup tomato sauce

Instructions
1. Press the Sauté button on the Instant Pot.
2. Heat the oil and sauté the onion and garlic.
3. Add in the beef stew meat and stir for another 3 minutes until lightly brown.
4. Stir in the rest of the ingredients. Mix well to combine.
5. Close the lid and press the Meat/Stew button.
6. Adjust the cooking time to 40 minutes.
7. Do natural pressure release.

Nutrition information:
Calories per serving: 411; Carbohydrates: 12.6g; Protein: 37.8g; Fat: 22.2g; Fiber: 3.2g

Instant Pot Nikujaga

Serves: 4
Preparation Time: 4 minutes
Cooking Time: 45 minutes

Ingredients
- 10 green beans, trimmed

- 1 onion, chopped
- 1 carrots, cubed
- 2 potatoes, cubed
- ½ pounds sliced beef chuck
- Salt

Instructions
1. Place all ingredients in the Instant Pot.
2. Close the lid and press the Meat/Stew button.
3. Adjust the cooking time to 45 minutes.
4. Do natural pressure release.

Nutrition information:
Calories per serving: 244; Carbohydrates: 36.9g; Protein: 16.4g; Fat: 3.9g; Fiber: 5.2g

Brazilian Beef Stew (Feijoada)

Serves: 8
Preparation Time: 5 minutes
Cooking Time: 40 minutes

Ingredients
- 4 tablespoons vegetable oil
- 1 onion, chopped
- 12 cloves of garlic, sliced
- 2 ½ pounds chuck stew meat
- Salt and pepper
- 2 poblano peppers, seeded and chopped
- 1 cup yellow squash, sliced
- 3 cups beef broth
- 1 cup tomatoes, chopped
- 2 tablespoons red wine vinegar
- 2 tablespoons chili powder
- 2 cans black beans, drained and rinsed

Instructions
1. Press the Sauté button on the Instant Pot.
2. Heat the oil and sauté the onion and garlic.
3. Add in the beef stew meat and stir for another 3 minutes until lightly brown.
4. Season with salt and pepper to taste.
5. Stir in the rest of the ingredients.
6. Close the lid and press the Meat/Stew button.
7. Adjust the cooking time to 40 minutes.
8. Do natural pressure release.
9. Serve with rice and lime wedges.

Nutrition information:
Calories per serving: 483; Carbohydrates: 24.4g; Protein: 40.8g; Fat: 24.4g; Fiber: 5.4g

Beef Barley Stew with Sour Cream

Serves: 4
Preparation Time: 4 minutes
Cooking Time: 40 minutes

Ingredients
- 1-pound beef stew meat, cut into small chunks
- 1 onion, chopped
- 1 cloves of garlic, minced
- 3 cups beef broth
- 1 cup mushrooms, sliced
- Salt and pepper
- 1 bay leaf
- 1 tablespoon thyme
- 1 tablespoon tomato paste
- ½ cup uncooked pearl barley
- ½ cup sour cream

Instructions
1. Place all ingredients in the Instant Pot.
2. Close the lid and press the Meat/Stew button.
3. Adjust the cooking time to 40 minutes.
4. Do natural pressure release.
5. Once the lid is open, press the Sauté button and add the sour cream.
6. Allow simmering for a few minutes.

Nutrition information:
Calories per serving: 309; Carbohydrates: 43.7g; Protein: 5.69g; Fat: 13.15g; Fiber: 5.5g

Instant Pot Mongolian Beef

Serves: 4
Preparation Time: 5 minutes
Cooking Time: 40 minutes

Ingredients
- 2 tablespoons olive oil
- 1 ½ pounds flank steak, sliced
- ½ teaspoon grated ginger
- ¾ cup coconut aminos
- ¾ cup water
- ¾ cup honey
- ½ cups grated carrots
- 1 tablespoon cornstarch + 2 tablespoons water

Instructions
1. Press the Sauté button on the Instant Pot.
2. Heat the oil and sauté the beef stew meat and stir for another 3 minutes until lightly brown.
3. Add the ginger, coconut aminos, water, honey, and carrots.
4. Close the lid and press the Meat/Stew button.
5. Adjust the cooking time to 40 minutes.
6. Do natural pressure release.
7. Once the lid is open, press the Sauté button and stir in the cornstarch slurry.
8. Allow simmering until the sauce thickens.

Nutrition information:
Calories per serving: 439; Carbohydrates: 41.9g; Protein: 45.9g; Fat: 9.5g; Fiber: 5g

Easy Beef and Broccoli Stir Fry

Serves: 5
Preparation Time: 5 minutes
Cooking Time: 25 minutes

Ingredients
- 1 tablespoon olive oil
- 1 onion, chopped
- 3 cloves of garlic, minced
- 1-pound flank steak, thinly sliced
- 1 tablespoon ginger, grated
- 1 tablespoon Shaoxing wine
- 2 tablespoons soy sauce
- ½ tablespoon oyster sauce
- 1/3 teaspoon five spice powder
- 1 cup beef broth
- ¼ teaspoon brown sugar
- 1 head broccoli, cut into florets

- 1 tablespoon cornstarch + 2 tablespoons water

Instructions
1. Press the Sauté button on the Instant Pot.
2. Heat the oil and sauté the onions and garlic until fragrant.
3. Stir in the beef stew meat and stir for another 3 minutes until lightly brown.
4. Add the rest of the ingredients except for the broccoli and cornstarch slurry.
5. Close the lid and press the Meat/Stew button.
6. Adjust the cooking time to 20 minutes.
7. Do natural pressure release.
8. Once the lid is open, press the Sauté button and stir in the broccoli and cornstarch slurry.
9. Allow simmering until the sauce thickens and the broccoli cooked.

Nutrition information:
Calories per serving: 500; Carbohydrates: 55.4g; Protein: 37.1g; Fat: 15.4g; Fiber: 1g

Instant Pot Beef Ragu

Serves: 4
Preparation Time: 3 minutes
Cooking Time: 30 minutes

Ingredients
- 2 tablespoons oil
- 1 onion, chopped
- 3 cloves of garlic
- 1 ½ pounds beef steak, cut into strips
- 1 bay leaf
- 1 teaspoon ground paprika
- 1 star anise
- 1 carrot, chopped
- 1 stalk of celery, minced
- ½ long red chili, chopped
- 1 cup beef broth
- 1 can crushed tomatoes
- Salt and pepper

Instructions
1. Press the Sauté button on the Instant Pot.
2. Heat the oil and sauté the onions and garlic until fragrant.
3. Stir in the beef stew meat and stir for another 3 minutes until lightly brown.
4. Add the rest of the ingredients.
5. Close the lid and press the Meat/Stew button.
6. Adjust the cooking time to 30 minutes.
7. Do natural pressure release.

Nutrition information:
Calories per serving: 356; Carbohydrates: 13.2g; Protein: 37.6g; Fat: 16.7g; Fiber: 2.4g

Italian Tomato Meatballs

Serves: 4
Preparation Time: 30 minutes
Cooking Time: 40 minutes

Ingredients
- 1 ¼ pounds ground beef
- 1 teaspoon onion powder
- 1 teaspoon garlic powder
- 1 teaspoon dried oregano
- ½ teaspoon celery salt
- 2 tablespoons olive oil
- 1 onion, diced
- 2 cloves garlic, minced
- 1 can chopped tomatoes
- Salt and pepper

Instructions
1. In a mixing bowl, combine the first 5 ingredients. Form small balls using your hands and set aside in the fridge for at least 30 minutes.
2. Press the Sauté button on the Instant Pot.
3. Heat the oil and sauté the onions and garlic until fragrant.
4. Add the meatballs and stir carefully until all sides have seared.
5. Pour in the rest of the ingredients.
6. Close the lid and press the Meat/Stew button.
7. Adjust the cooking time to 35 minutes.
8. Do natural pressure release.

Nutrition information:
Calories per serving: 451; Carbohydrates: 7.1g; Protein: 36.9g; Fat: 29.8g; Fiber: 1.9g

Instant Pot Sloppy Joes

Serves: 8
Preparation Time: 4 minutes
Cooking Time: 40 minutes

Ingredients
- 1 tablespoon oil
- 1 onion, chopped
- 3 cloves of garlic, minced
- 1-pound ground beef
- 1 green red bell pepper, chopped
- 1 carrot, grated
- Salt and pepper
- 1 tablespoons Worcestershire sauce
- 4 tablespoons apple cider vinegar
- 1 cup chopped tomatoes
- 4 tablespoons tomato paste
- 1 cup water

Instructions
1. Press the Sauté button on the Instant Pot.
2. Heat the oil and sauté the onions and garlic until fragrant.
3. Stir in the ground beef and keep on stirring for 5 minutes.
4. Pour in the rest of the ingredients.
5. Close the lid and press the Meat/Stew button.
6. Adjust the cooking time to 35 minutes.
7. Do natural pressure release.

Nutrition information:
Calories per serving: 180; Carbohydrates: 18g; Protein: 15g; Fat: 5.8g; Fiber: 3.6 g

Korean Basil Beef Bowls

Serves: 4
Preparation Time: 5 minutes
Cooking Time: 40 minutes

Ingredients

- 1 tablespoon oil
- 1 onion, chopped
- 5 cloves of garlic, minced
- 1-pound ground beef
- 1 tablespoon ginger, julienned
- 2 dried red chilies
- Salt and pepper
- 1 cup fresh basil, chopped
- ¼ cup chicken broth
- 1 tablespoon soy sauce
- 1 teaspoon sugar
- 2 tablespoons gochujang paste
- 1 tablespoon sesame oil

Instructions
1. Press the Sauté button on the Instant Pot.
2. Heat the oil and sauté the onions and garlic until fragrant.
3. Stir in the ground beef and keep on stirring for 5 minutes.
4. Add the rest of the ingredients.
5. Close the lid and press the Meat/Stew button.
6. Adjust the cooking time to 35 minutes.
7. Do natural pressure release.

Nutrition information:
Calories per serving: 416; Carbohydrates: 8.6g; Protein: 33.4g; Fat: 27.1g; Fiber: 1.3g

Corned Beef Brisket

Serves: 9
Preparation Time: 5 minutes
Cooking Time: 1 hour and 15 minutes

Ingredients
- 3 pounds corned beef brisket
- 1 onion, chopped
- 3 cloves of garlic
- 1 ½ cups dark ale
- 2 potatoes, cubed
- 2 carrots, cubed

Instructions
1. Place all ingredients in the Instant Pot.
2. Close the lid and press the Meat/Stew button.
3. Adjust the cooking time to 1 hour and 30 minutes.
4. Do natural pressure release.

Nutrition information:
Calories per serving: 388; Carbohydrates: 20.8g; Protein: 28.2g; Fat: 24.3g; Fiber: 2.4g

Pork Recipes

Instant Pot Ribs
Serves: 4
Preparation Time: 3 minutes
Cooking Time: 30 minutes
Ingredients
- ½ rack spare ribs
- Salt and pepper
- 1 cup beef stock
- 3 tablespoons Dijon mustard
- 3 tablespoons brown sugar

Instructions
1. Place all ingredients in the Instant Pot.
2. Close the lid and press the Meat/Stew button.
3. Adjust the cooking time to 30 minutes.
4. Do natural pressure release.

Nutrition information:
Calories per serving: 140; Carbohydrates: 6.9g; Protein: 17.1g; Fat: 4.6g; Fiber: 0.7g

Smoky BBQ Instant Pot Ribs
Serves: 8
Preparation Time: 4 minutes
Cooking Time: 40 minutes
Ingredients
- 2 pounds spare ribs
- 1 can chicken broth
- 1 tablespoon liquid smoke
- 1 cup BBQ sauce
- Salt and pepper

Instructions
1. Place all ingredients in the Instant Pot.
2. Close the lid and press the Meat/Stew button.
3. Adjust the cooking time to 40 minutes.
4. Do natural pressure release.

Nutrition information:
Calories per serving: 400; Carbohydrates: 5.4g; Protein: 55.8g; Fat: 15.7g; Fiber: 1.4g

Sticky Glazed Spare Ribs
Serves: 4
Preparation Time: 3 minutes
Cooking Time: 40 minutes
Ingredients
- 6 tablespoons black currant jelly
- 2 tablespoons honey
- 2 cloves of garlic, minced
- 1 tablespoon grated ginger
- 1 tablespoon chili, minced
- 2 tablespoons soy sauce
- 2 pounds spare ribs

Instructions
1. Place all ingredients in the Instant Pot.
2. Close the lid and press the Meat/Stew button.
3. Adjust the cooking time to 40 minutes.
4. Do natural pressure release.

Nutrition information:
Calories per serving: 356; Carbohydrates: 5.5g; Protein: 48.9g; Fat: 14.5g; Fiber: 0.9g

Coffee Pork Ribs
Serves: 4
Preparation Time: 3 minutes
Cooking Time: 40 minutes
Ingredients
- 1 rack baby back ribs
- 2 teaspoons sesame oil
- 3 tablespoons oyster sauce
- 1 teaspoon salt
- 1 teaspoon sugar
- 1 cup water
- ½ cup liquid smoke
- 2 tablespoons instant coffee powder

Instructions
1. Place all ingredients in the Instant Pot.
2. Close the lid and press the Meat/Stew button.
3. Adjust the cooking time to 40 minutes.
4. Do natural pressure release.

Nutrition information:
Calories per serving: 898; Carbohydrates: 4.1g; Protein: 77.3g; Fat: 63.7g; Fiber: 0g

Instant Pot Korean Glazed Ribs
Serves: 8
Preparation Time: 4 minutes
Cooking Time: 45 minutes
Ingredients
- 2-pound baby back ribs, cut into single ribs
- 2 cloves of garlic, minced
- 1 teaspoon onion powder
- ¾ cup soy sauce
- ¾ cup brown sugar
- 1 cup chicken broth
- 1 tablespoon sesame oil
- Salt and pepper

Instructions
1. Place all ingredients in the Instant Pot.
2. Close the lid and press the Meat/Stew button.
3. Adjust the cooking time to 45 minutes.
4. Do natural pressure release.

Nutrition information:
Calories per serving: 465; Carbohydrates: 27.6g; Protein: 30.7g; Fat: 25.9g; Fiber: 0.7g

Maple Spice Rubbed Ribs
Serves: 4
Preparation Time: 4 minutes
Cooking Time: 45 minutes
Ingredients
- 3 tablespoons chili powder, divided
- 1 ¼ teaspoon ground coriander
- 1 ¼ teaspoon garlic powder
- Salt and pepper
- 3 ½ pounds baby back ribs
- 4 tablespoons maple syrup
- 1 can tomato sauce
- ¼ teaspoon ground cinnamon
- ¼ teaspoon ground ginger

Instructions
1. Place all ingredients in the Instant Pot.
2. Close the lid and press the Meat/Stew button.
3. Adjust the cooking time to 45 minutes.
4. Do natural pressure release.

Nutrition information:
Calories per serving:955; Carbohydrates: 19.2g; Protein: 79.4g; Fat: 63.5g; Fiber: 3.5g

Sweet and Sour Riblets

Serves: 5
Preparation Time: 4 minutes
Cooking Time: 40 minutes
Ingredients
- 1 cup pineapple juice
- 1/3 cup packed brown sugar
- 1/3 cup rice vinegar
- 3 tablespoons ketchup
- 2 tablespoons soy sauce
- 1 rack of rib
- Salt and pepper
- 1 tablespoon cornstarch + 2 tablespoons water

Instructions
1. Place all ingredients in the Instant Pot.
2. Close the lid and press the Meat/Stew button.
3. Adjust the cooking time to 40 minutes.
4. Do natural pressure release.

Nutrition information:
Calories per serving: 176; Carbohydrates: 27.8g; Protein: 9.1g; Fat: 3.4g; Fiber: 0.7g

Fall-Of-The-Bones Ribs

Serves: 8
Preparation Time: 5 minutes
Cooking Time: 60 minutes
Ingredients
- 2 racks of ribs
- 2 cups apple juice
- 1 can light beer
- 1 cup BBQ sauce

Instructions
1. Place all ingredients in the Instant Pot.
2. Close the lid and press the Meat/Stew button.
3. Adjust the cooking time to 60 minutes.
4. Do natural pressure release.

Nutrition information:
Calories per serving: 113; Carbohydrates: 10.4g; Protein: 10.9g; Fat: 3.1g; Fiber: 0.7g

Greek Pork Ribs

Serves: 6
Preparation Time: 4 minutes
Cooking Time: 40 minutes
Ingredients
- 2 racks of baby back or spare ribs
- 1 tablespoon oil
- Juice of 2 lemons
- 2 teaspoons salt
- 1 teaspoon pepper
- 2 teaspoons smoked paprika
- 1 cup water

Instructions
1. Place all ingredients in the Instant Pot.
2. Close the lid and press the Meat/Stew button.
3. Adjust the cooking time to 40 minutes.
4. Do natural pressure release.

Nutrition information:
Calories per serving: 549; Carbohydrates: 10.6g; Protein: 48.5g; Fat: 10.4g; Fiber: 3g

Instant Pot Barbecue Ribs

Serves: 4
Preparation Time: 5 minutes
Cooking Time: 40 minutes
Ingredients
- 2 racks of pork ribs
- 1 cup apple juice
- ½ teaspoon liquid smoke
- 6 fresh sage leaves
- ½ onion, chopped
- 1 cup BBQ sauce
- Salt and pepper

Instructions
1. Place all ingredients in the Instant Pot.
2. Close the lid and press the Meat/Stew button.
3. Adjust the cooking time to 40 minutes.
4. Do natural pressure release.

Nutrition information:
Calories per serving: 196; Carbohydrates: 13.7g; Protein: 21.8g; Fat: 5.8g; Fiber: 1.7g

Instant Pot Kalua Pig

Serves: 8
Preparation Time: 5 minutes
Cooking Time: 40 minutes
Ingredients
- 3 bacon slices
- 5-pound bone-in pork shoulder roast
- 5 cloves of garlic, minced
- 1 cup water
- 1 cabbage, cut into wedges

Instructions
1. Press the Sauté button on the Instant Pot.
2. Add the bacon slices and cook until crisp. Set aside.
3. Stir in the pork shoulder roasts and garlic. Stir to sear all sides.
4. Add the water and close the lid.
5. Press the Manual button and adjust the cooking time to 45 minutes.
6. Do quick pressure release.
7. Once the lid is open, press the Sauté button.
8. Put the cabbages and simmer for 5 minutes.

Nutrition information:
Calories per serving: 730; Carbohydrates: 11.2g; Protein: 86.5g; Fat: 36.3g; Fiber: 3g

Western Shoulder Ribs

Serves: 8
Preparation Time: 5 minutes
Cooking Time: 40 minutes
Ingredients
- 3 pounds pork shoulder
- 2 teaspoons salt
- 1 teaspoon barbecue rub
- ½ cup water
- ½ cup commercial barbecue sauce

Instructions
1. Place all ingredients in the Instant Pot.
2. Close the lid and press the Meat/Stew button.
3. Adjust the cooking time to 40 minutes.

4. Do natural pressure release.
Nutrition information:
Calories per serving: 470; Carbohydrates: 2.8g; Protein: 43.7g; Fat: 30.1g; Fiber: 0g

Pork Ribs with Memphis Rub
Serves: 4
Preparation Time: 5 minutes
Cooking Time: 60 minutes
Ingredients
- 3 pounds baby back ribs
- ½ cup water
- 1 cup ketchup
- 1 cup tomato sauce
- ½ cup apple cider vinegar
- 2 tablespoon light brown sugar
- ½ tablespoons ground black pepper
- 2 tablespoon molasses
- 1 teaspoon onion powder
- 1 teaspoon garlic powder
- 1 tablespoon Dijon mustard
- 1 tablespoon Worcestershire sauce
- ¼ cup paprika
- 1 ½ teaspoon cumin

Instructions
1. Place all ingredients in the Instant Pot.
2. Close the lid and press the Meat/Stew button.
3. Adjust the cooking time to 60 minutes.
4. Do natural pressure release.

Nutrition information:
Calories per serving: 825; Carbohydrates: 4.2g; Protein: 68g; Fat: 32g; Fiber: 0.9g

Instant Pot Paleo Carnitas
Serves: 9
Preparation Time: 5 minutes
Cooking Time: 60 minutes
Ingredients
- 3 pounds pork butt
- 1 tablespoons dried oregano
- 1 teaspoon cinnamon
- ½ teaspoon ground cloves
- 2 dried bay leaves
- 4 cloves of garlic
- 1 onion, chopped
- ½ cup water
- Juice of 1 lemon, freshly squeezed

Instructions
1. Place all ingredients in the Instant Pot.
2. Close the lid and press the Meat/Stew button.
3. Adjust the cooking time to 60 minutes.
4. Do natural pressure release.
5. Once the lid is open, take the pork out and use two forks to shred the meat.
6. Serve with the sauce.

Nutrition information:
Calories per serving: 412; Carbohydrates: 2.8g; Protein: 38.6g; Fat: 26.7g; Fiber: 0.4g

Smoked Pull Pork
Serves: 12
Preparation Time: 5 minutes
Cooking Time: 60 minutes
Ingredients
- 3 ½ pounds pork butt roast
- 1 cup chicken broth
- 2 tablespoons soy sauce
- 2 tablespoons liquid smoke
- 2 cloves of garlic, minced

Instructions
1. Place all ingredients in the Instant Pot.
2. Close the lid and press the Meat/Stew button.
3. Adjust the cooking time to 60 minutes.
4. Do natural pressure release.
5. Once the lid is open, take the pork out and use two forks to shred the meat.
6. Serve with the sauce.

Nutrition information:
Calories per serving: 392; Carbohydrates: 0.5 g; Protein: 31.4g; Fat: 28.4g; Fiber: 0g

BBQ Pulled Pork
Serves: 9
Preparation Time: 5 minutes
Cooking Time: 60 minutes
Ingredients
- ½ cup BBQ sauce
- ½ cup chicken broth
- 3 pounds pork roast
- Salt and pepper

Instructions
1. Place all ingredients in the Instant Pot.
2. Close the lid and press the Meat/Stew button.
3. Adjust the cooking time to 60 minutes.
4. Do natural pressure release.
5. Once the lid is open, take the pork out and use two forks to shred the meat.
6. Serve with the sauce.

Nutrition information:
Calories per serving: 318; Carbohydrates: 1.6g; Protein: 43.1g; Fat: 14.5g; Fiber: 0.4g

Orange-Glazed Pork Chops
Serves: 4
Preparation Time: 5 minutes
Cooking Time: 30 minutes
Ingredients
- 4 pork chops
- Salt and pepper
- 1 tablespoons olive oil
- 1 cup chicken broth
- 1 teaspoon orange zest
- ¼ teaspoon dried thyme
- ¼ teaspoon onion powder
- ½ cup orange marmalade
- 1 tablespoon apple cider vinegar
- 2 tablespoons soy sauce

Instructions
1. Season the pork chops with salt and pepper to taste.
2. Press the Sauté button on the Instant Pot.
3. Heat the oil and place the pork chops.
4. Sear on all sides.
5. Add the rest of the ingredients.
6. Close the lid and press the Meat/Stew button.
7. Adjust the cooking time to 30 minutes.

8. Do natural pressure release.
Nutrition information:
Calories per serving: 582; Carbohydrates: 30.8g; Protein: 54.6g; Fat: 26.8g; Fiber: 0.7g

Buffalo Pork Chops
Serves: 2
Preparation Time:
Cooking Time: 20 minutes
Ingredients
- 2 tablespoons oil
- 2 boneless pork chops
- 2 tablespoons butter
- 2 tablespoons hot sauce
- 1 cup water
- ½ cup mozzarella cheese, grated

Instructions
1. Press the Sauté button on the Instant Pot.
2. Heat the oil and place the pork chops.
3. Sear on all sides.
4. Stir in the butter, hot sauce, and water. Stir.
5. Sprinkle with mozzarella cheese on top.
6. Close the lid and press the Meat/Stew button.
7. Adjust the cooking time to 20 minutes.
8. Do natural pressure release.

Nutrition information:
Calories per serving: 498; Carbohydrates: 1.5g; Protein: 50.6g; Fat: 31.5g; Fiber: 0.6g

Honey Lime Ginger Pork Chops
Serves: 5
Preparation Time: 5 minutes
Cooking Time: 25 minutes
Ingredients
- ½ cup honey
- ¼ cup soy sauce
- 1 tablespoon Worcestershire sauce
- Juice of 1 lime
- 2 cloves of garlic, minced
- 1 teaspoon ginger, ground
- 5 pork chops
- Salt and pepper
- 1 tablespoon olive oil
- 1 cup water
- 1 tablespoon cornstarch + 2 tablespoons water

Instructions
1. In a mixing bowl, combine the first 6 ingredients. This will be the honey-lime mixture. Set aside.
2. Season the pork chops with salt and pepper to taste
3. Press the Sauté button on the Instant Pot.
4. Heat the oil and place the pork chops.
5. Sear on all sides.
6. Pour honey lime mixture prepared earlier over the pork.
7. Stir in water.
8. Close the lid and press the Meat/Stew button.
9. Adjust the cooking time to 20 minutes.
10. Do quick pressure release.
11. Once the lid is open, press the Sauté button and stir in the cornstarch slurry.
12. Allow simmering until the sauce thickens.

Nutrition information:
Calories per serving: 503; Carbohydrates: 33.8g; Protein: 41.7g; Fat: 22.4g; Fiber: 0.6g

Instant Pot Pork Adobo
Serves: 9
Preparation Time: 3 minutes
Cooking Time: 30 minutes
Ingredients
- 3 pounds pork butt, cut into cubes
- 2 bay leaves
- ½ cup soy sauce
- ¼ cup rice vinegar
- 1 teaspoon whole black peppercorns
- 3 tablespoons brown sugar
- 5 cloves of garlic, crushed
- 1 onion, chopped

Instructions
1. Place all ingredients in the Instant Pot.
2. Close the lid and press the Meat/Stew button.
3. Adjust the cooking time to 30 minutes.
4. Do natural pressure release.

Nutrition information:
Calories per serving: 454; Carbohydrates: 5.3g; Protein: 39.7g; Fat: 29.5g; Fiber: 0.5g

Instant Pot Curried Pork Chops
Serves: 2
Preparation Time: 5 minutes
Cooking Time: 30 minutes
Ingredients
- 2 pork chops
- 4 carrots, chopped
- 4 small potatoes, cubed
- 2 cloves of garlic, minced
- ¼ cup balsamic vinegar
- ¼ cup soy sauce
- 2 tablespoons honey
- 2 teaspoons grated ginger
- 2 teaspoons curry powder
- ½ cup chicken stock
- Salt and pepper

Instructions
1. Place all ingredients in the Instant Pot.
2. Close the lid and press the Meat/Stew button.
3. Adjust the cooking time to 30 minutes.
4. Do natural pressure release.

Nutrition information:
Calories per serving: 1175; Carbohydrates: 178g; Protein: 61g; Fat: 25.9g; Fiber: 21.1g

Pork Chops with Honey Mustard
Serves: 4
Preparation Time: 5 minutes
Cooking Time: 30 minutes
Ingredients
- 1 tablespoon olive oil
- 4 pork chops
- ½ cup onions, sliced
- 3 tablespoons garlic, minced
- 8 ounces white button mushrooms, sliced
- 4 cups green beans, chopped
- 2 cups chicken broth
- ¼ cup honey

- ½ cup Dijon mustard
- Salt and pepper
- 1 tablespoon cornstarch + 2 tablespoons water

Instructions
1. Press the Sauté button on the Instant Pot.
2. Heat the oil and place the pork chops. Sear on all sides.
3. Stir in the onions and garlic until fragrant.
4. Add the remaining ingredients except for the cornstarch slurry.
5. Close the lid and press the Meat/Stew button.
6. Adjust the cooking time to 30 minutes.
7. Do natural pressure release.

Nutrition information:
Calories per serving:370; Carbohydrates: 7g; Protein: 27g; Fat: 12g; Fiber: 3.6g

Smothered Pork Chops

Serves: 4
Preparation Time: 5 minutes
Cooking Time: 30 minutes

Ingredients
- 1 onion, diced
- 2 cloves of garlic, minced
- ½ teaspoon dried thyme
- ½ teaspoon brown sugar
- ½ cup chicken broth
- 2 tablespoons soy sauce
- 1-pound thin sirloin pork chops
- Salt and pepper
- 1 ½ teaspoon apple cider vinegar
- 2 tablespoons cornstarch + 3 tablespoons water

Instructions
1. Place all ingredients in the Instant Pot except for the cornstarch slurry.
2. Close the lid and press the Meat/Stew button.
3. Adjust the cooking time to 30 minutes.
4. Do natural pressure release.
5. Once the lid is open, press the Sauté button.
6. Stir in the cornstarch slurry and allow to simmer until the sauce thickens.

Nutrition information:
Calories per serving: 229; Carbohydrates: 7.2g; Protein: 33.4g; Fat: 6.5g; Fiber:0.9g

Chili Verde Recipe

Serves: 10
Preparation Time: 5 minutes
Cooking Time: 30 minutes

Ingredients
- 4 pounds sirloin pork roast, cut into cubes
- 2 onions, chopped
- 3 cloves of garlic, minced
- 1-pound tomatillos
- 5 cloves of garlic, minced
- 2 chili peppers
- 1 tablespoon dried oregano
- 1 teaspoon cumin
- 1 bunch cilantro leaves, chopped
- 2 ½ cups chicken stock
- Salt and pepper

Instructions
1. Place all ingredients in the Instant Pot.
2. Close the lid and press the Meat/Stew button.
3. Adjust the cooking time to 30 minutes.
4. Do natural pressure release.
5. Serve with cheese if desired.

Nutrition information:
Calories per serving:260; Carbohydrates: 9.1g; Protein: 44.1g; Fat: 4.4g; Fiber: 1.5g

Instant Pot Pineapple Ham

Serves: 6
Preparation Time: 5 minutes
Cooking Time: 30 minutes

Ingredients
- 1 frozen ham
- 1 can crushed pineapples
- ¼ cup dark brown sugar
- ½ cups water

Instructions
1. Place all ingredients in the Instant Pot.
2. Close the lid and press the Meat/Stew button.
3. Adjust the cooking time to 30 minutes.
4. Do natural pressure release.

Nutrition information:
Calories per serving:158; Carbohydrates: 20.8g; Protein: 13.2g; Fat:2.6 g; Fiber: 0.3g

Beer-Braised Pulled Ham

Serves: 16
Preparation Time: 5 minutes
Cooking Time: 60 minutes

Ingredients
- 2 bottles of beer
- ¾ cup Dijon mustard
- ½ teaspoon ground black pepper
- 1 bone-in ham
- 4 sprigs of rosemary

Instructions
1. Place all ingredients in the Instant Pot.
2. Close the lid and press the Meat/Stew button.
3. Adjust the cooking time to 60 minutes.
4. Do natural pressure release.
5. Take the pork out and use two forks to shred the meat.

Nutrition information:
Calories per serving: 56; Carbohydrates: 2.7g; Protein: 5.6g; Fat:1.4g; Fiber: 0.5g

Cranberry Maple Orange Pork Chops

Serves: 5
Preparation Time: 5 minutes
Cooking Time: 30 minutes

Ingredients
- 4 tablespoons coconut oil
- 1 ½ pounds pork chop, bone in
- 1 onion, diced
- ½ cup orange juice
- ¼ cup maple syrup
- 1 ½ teaspoon cinnamon
- 1 teaspoon garlic cloves
- 1/3 cup cranberries
- 2 teaspoons rosemary, fresh
- Salt and pepper

Instructions

1. Press the Sauté button on the Instant Pot.
2. Heat the oil and place the pork chops. Sear on all sides.
3. Stir in the rest of the ingredients. Scrape the bottom to remove the browning.
4. Close the lid and press the Meat/Stew button.
5. Adjust the cooking time to 60 minutes.
6. Do natural pressure release.

Nutrition information:
Calories per serving:388; Carbohydrates: 3.2g; Protein: 45g; Fat: 29g; Fiber: 0.7g

3-Ingredient Pork Chops

Serves: 2
Preparation Time: 5 minutes
Cooking Time: 25 minutes

Ingredients
- 2 tablespoons lemon pepper
- 2 pork chops, bone in
- ¼ cup apple juice

Instructions
1. Place all ingredients in the Instant Pot.
2. Close the lid and press the Meat/Stew button.
3. Adjust the cooking time to 25 minutes.
4. Do natural pressure release.

Nutrition information:
Calories per serving: 342; Carbohydrates:3.5 g; Protein: 40.3g; Fat: 17.4g; Fiber: 0.1g

Shortcut Pork Posole

Serves: 4
Preparation Time: 5 minutes
Cooking Time: 30 minutes

Ingredients
- 1-pound pork shoulder, cut into chunks
- 1 onion, chopped
- 4 cloves of garlic, minced
- 25 ounces posole
- 1 can chipotle chilies
- 1 teaspoon dried oregano
- 2 teaspoon ground cumin
- ¾ cup water
- ¼ cup cilantro, chopped

Instructions
1. Place all ingredients in the Instant Pot.
2. Close the lid and press the Meat/Stew button.
3. Adjust the cooking time to 30 minutes.
4. Do natural pressure release.

Nutrition information:
Calories per serving:391; Carbohydrates: 8.3g; Protein: 72g; Fat: 3g; Fiber: 3.4g

Moo Shu Pork

Serves: 4
Preparation Time: 5 minutes
Cooking Time: 30 minutes

Ingredients
- 2 teaspoon sesame oil
- 1 onion, chopped
- 1 tablespoon minced garlic
- 1-pound pork chops, cut into strips
- ¼ cup beef broth
- 3 tablespoon soy sauce
- 1/3 cup hoisin sauce
- 1 bag of shredded cabbages
- 2 tablespoon cornstarch + 2 tablespoons water

Instructions
1. Press the Sauté button on the Instant Pot.
2. Heat the oil and sauté the onion and garlic until fragrant.
3. Add in the pork strips and sauté for 5 minutes.
4. Pour in the broth, soy sauce, and hoisin sauce.
5. Close the lid and press the Meat/Stew button.
6. Adjust the cooking time to 25 minutes.
7. Do natural pressure release.
8. Once the lid is open, stir in the shredded cabbages and cornstarch slurry.
9. Allow simmering until the sauce thickens.

Nutrition information:
Calories per serving: 363; Carbohydrates:18.2 g; Protein: 31.5g; Fat: 17.6g; Fiber: 1.7g

Instant Pot Asian Pork Belly

Serves: 9
Preparation Time: 5 minutes
Cooking Time: 45 minutes

Ingredients
- 3 pounds pork belly
- 1 thumb-size ginger, sliced thinly
- 3 stalks of green onions, chopped
- 4 cloves of garlic, minced
- 4 star anise
- 4 cloves
- ½ cup brown sugar
- ½ cup soy sauce
- ½ cup soy paste
- ½ cup Shaoxing wine

Instructions
1. Place all ingredients in the Instant Pot.
2. Close the lid and press the Meat/Stew button.
3. Adjust the cooking time to 45 minutes.
4. Do natural pressure release.

Nutrition information:
Calories per serving: 882; Carbohydrates: 16.9g; Protein: 16.5g; Fat: 82.7g; Fiber: 0.4g

Instant Pot Pork Stroganoff

Serves: 4
Preparation Time: 5 minutes
Cooking Time: 40 minutes

Ingredients
- 1-pound pork loin, cut into strips
- 3 carrots, chopped
- 2 stalks of celery, chopped
- 1 onion, chopped
- 1 tablespoon Dijon mustard
- ½ cup sour cream
- 2 cups chicken broth
- 1 package egg noodles, cooked

Instructions
1. Place all ingredients except for the cooked egg noodles in the Instant Pot.
2. Close the lid and press the Meat/Stew button.
3. Adjust the cooking time to 40 minutes.
4. Do natural pressure release.
5. Serve on top of cooked egg noodles

Nutrition information:
Calories per serving:602; Carbohydrates: 16g; Protein: 85g; Fat: 19g; Fiber: 1g

Hungarian Pork Paprikash

Serves: 6
Preparation Time: 4 minutes
Cooking Time: 40 minutes
Ingredients
- 4 pounds pork loin
- 1 onion, chopped
- 1 cup mushrooms, sliced
- ¼ cup chicken stock
- ¼ cup red wine vinegar
- 6 ounces tomato paste
- 3 cloves of garlic, minced
- 5 tablespoons Hungarian sweet paprika, sliced
- ¼ cup basil leaves
- ¾ cup sour cream

Instructions
1. Place all ingredients in the Instant Pot.
2. Close the lid and press the Meat/Stew button.
3. Adjust the cooking time to 40 minutes.
4. Do natural pressure release.

Nutrition information:
Calories per serving: 726; Carbohydrates: 13.1g; Protein: 81.6g; Fat: 37.5g; Fiber: 3.5g

Simple General Tso's Pork

Serves: 5
Preparation Time: 5 minutes
Cooking Time: 40 minutes
Ingredients
- 1 ½ tablespoons rice vinegar
- 2 tablespoons rice wine
- 3 tablespoons sugar
- 3 tablespoons soy sauce
- 1-pound pork tenderloin
- 1 cup chicken broth
- 1 dried chili pods, chopped
- 1 onion, chopped
- 1 tablespoon cornstarch + 2 tablespoons water

Instructions
1. Place all ingredients in the Instant Pot.
2. Close the lid and press the Meat/Stew button.
3. Adjust the cooking time to 40 minutes.
4. Do natural pressure release.

Nutrition information:
Calories per serving: 271; Carbohydrates: 11.1g; Protein: 35.4g; Fat: 9.9g; Fiber: 1.2g

Peppercorn Pork Brisket

Serves: 12
Preparation Time: 5 minutes
Cooking Time: 40 minutes
Ingredients
- 4 pounds pork brisket
- 3 tablespoons peppercorn
- 3 cloves of garlic, minced
- 2 cups red wine
- 2 cups chicken broth
- 1 tablespoon butter
- 1 cup mushrooms, sliced
- Salt and pepper

Instructions
1. Place all ingredients in the Instant Pot.
2. Close the lid and press the Meat/Stew button.
3. Adjust the cooking time to 40 minutes.
4. Do natural pressure release.

Nutrition information:
Calories per serving: 505; Carbohydrates: 1.1g; Protein: 46.7g; Fat: 32.5g; Fiber:0.1g

Ginger Pork Shogayaki

Serves: 4
Preparation Time: 5 minutes
Cooking Time: 40 minutes
Ingredients
- 1 tablespoon peanut oil
- 1-pound pork shoulder
- 1 onion, chopped
- 1 clove of garlic, minced
- Salt and pepper
- 1 thumb-size gingers, sliced
- 1 tablespoon soy sauce
- ½ teaspoon white miso paste
- 2 tablespoons cooking sake
- 2 tablespoons mirin
- ¼ cup water

Instructions
1. Press the Sauté button on the Instant Pot.
2. Heat the oil and sear the pork shoulder on all sides.
3. Stir in the onion and garlic. Season with salt and pepper.
4. Add the rest of the ingredients.
5. Close the lid and press the Meat/Stew button.
6. Adjust the cooking time to 40 minutes.
7. Do natural pressure release.

Nutrition information:
Calories per serving: 373; Carbohydrates: 5.5g; Protein: 29.6g; Fat: 24.7g; Fiber: 0.8g

Chile Pork Stew

Serves: 16
Preparation Time: 5 minutes
Cooking Time: 40 minutes
Ingredients
- 4 pounds pork loin roast, cut into 6 pieces
- 3 cans diced green chilies
- 3 poblano peppers, chopped
- 1 onion, diced
- 2 tablespoons chili powder
- 1 tablespoon paprika
- ¾ cup water
- Salt and pepper
- Cilantro, chopped

Instructions
1. Place all ingredients except for the cilantro in the Instant Pot.
2. Close the lid and press the Meat/Stew button.
3. Adjust the cooking time to 40 minutes.
4. Do natural pressure release.

Nutrition information:
Calories per serving: 229; Carbohydrates: 2.4g; Protein: 30.4g; Fat: 10.3g; Fiber: 0.8g

Chinese BBQ Pork (Char Siu)

Serves: 4
Preparation Time: 5 minutes
Cooking Time: 45 minutes

Ingredients
- 1-pound pork butt meat,
- 3 tablespoons honey
- 2 tablespoons soy sauce
- 1 cup water
- 1 tablespoon miso paste
- 3 tablespoons char siu sauce
- ½ teaspoon sesame oil
- 2 tablespoons Shaoxing wine
- Salt and pepper

Instructions
1. Place all ingredients except for the cilantro in the Instant Pot.
2. Close the lid and press the Meat/Stew button.
3. Adjust the cooking time to 45 minutes.
4. Do natural pressure release.

Nutrition information:
Calories per serving: 396; Carbohydrates: 18.9g; Protein: 29.4g; Fat: 22.6g; Fiber: 0.9g

Balsamic Spiced Apple Pork

Serves: 8
Preparation Time: 5 minutes
Cooking Time: 45 minutes

Ingredients
- 3 pounds pork tenderloins
- 3 granny smith apples, sliced
- ½ cup apple cider vinegar
- 1 tablespoon grapeseed oil
- 1 cinnamon stick
- 2 tablespoons butter
- 1 cup balsamic vinegar
- 2 tablespoon brown sugar
- 1 tablespoon orange zest
- Salt and pepper

Instructions
1. Place all ingredients except for the cilantro in the Instant Pot.
2. Close the lid and press the Meat/Stew button.
3. Adjust the cooking time to 45 minutes.
4. Do natural pressure release.

Nutrition information:
Calories per serving: 359; Carbohydrates: 16.4g; Protein: 45.9g; Fat: 10.7g; Fiber: 1.9g

Sweet Chili Sauce Braised Pork

Serves: 4
Preparation Time: 5 minutes
Cooking Time: 45 minutes

Ingredients
- 1 tablespoon vegetable oil
- 1 onion, chopped
- 1-pound pork shoulder, cut into large chunks
- ½ cup white sugar
- ½ cup water
- 3 tablespoons sweet chili sauce
- 3 cloves of garlic, minced
- 1 tablespoon sesame oil
- 1 tablespoon fish sauce
- 1 tablespoon hoisin sauce
- 1 teaspoon ground ginger

Instructions
1. Press the Sauté button on the Instant Pot.
2. Stir in the vegetable oil and sauté the onion.
3. Add in the pork shoulder. Stir for 3 minutes until the pork has turned golden.
4. Pour in the rest of the ingredients.
5. Close the lid and press the Meat/Stew button.
6. Adjust the cooking time to 45 minutes.
7. Do natural pressure release.

Nutrition information:
Calories per serving:457; Carbohydrates: 11.4g; Protein: 30.7g; Fat: 31.8g; Fiber:2.1g

Vegetables and Sides Recipes

Instant Pot Cauliflower Soup

Serves: 4
Preparation Time: 2 minutes
Cooking Time: 4 minutes
Ingredients
- 1 tablespoon butter
- ½ cup chopped onions
- 1 medium cauliflower, chopped
- 3 cups chicken broth
- Salt and pepper to taste

Instructions
1. Press the Sauté button on the Instant Pot.
2. Heat the butter and sauté the onions.
3. Add the rest of the ingredients.
4. Close the lid and press the Manual button.
5. Adjust the cooking time to 4 minutes.
6. Do quick pressure release.
7. Once the lid is open, place in a blender and puree until smooth.

Nutrition information:
Calories per serving:80; Carbohydrates: 11g; Protein: 6g; Fat: 3g; Fiber:4 g

Instant Pot Cauliflower Curry

Serves: 4
Preparation Time: 2 minutes
Cooking Time: 4 minutes
Ingredients
- 2 cups cauliflower florets
- 2 tablespoon garam masala
- 1 can full-fat coconut milk
- 2 cups water
- Salt and pepper to taste

Instructions
1. Place all ingredients in the Instant Pot.
2. Stir the contents and close the lid.
3. Close the lid and press the Manual button.
4. Adjust the cooking time to 4 minutes.
5. Do quick pressure release.

Nutrition information:
Calories per serving: 235; Carbohydrates: 35g; Protein: 21g; Fat: 10.5g; Fiber: 13g

Curried Squash Stew

Serves: 10
Preparation Time: 2 minutes
Cooking Time: 10 minutes
Ingredients
- 2 cups squash, chopped
- 1 can full-fat coconut milk
- 2 tablespoon garam masala
- Salt and pepper to taste
- 1 bag baby spinach, rinsed

Instructions
1. Place all ingredients except for the spinach in the Instant Pot.
2. Stir the contents and close the lid.
3. Close the lid and press the Manual button.
4. Adjust the cooking time to 10 minutes.
5. Do quick pressure release.
6. Once the lid is open, press the Sauté button.
7. Add the spinach and continue cooking until the greens have wilted.

Nutrition information:
Calories per serving: 123; Carbohydrates:1.78 g; Protein: 8.86g; Fat: 9.2g; Fiber: 1.5g

Vegan Pumpkin Stew

Serves: 4
Preparation Time: 3 minutes
Cooking Time: 10 minutes
Ingredients
- 3 cups pumpkin, sliced
- 5 cups vegetable stock
- 1 large can diced tomatoes
- Salt and pepper to taste
- 3 cups of mixed greens

Instructions
1. Place all ingredients in the Instant Pot.
2. Stir the contents and close the lid.
3. Close the lid and press the Manual button.
4. Adjust the cooking time to 10 minutes.
5. Do quick pressure release.

Nutrition information:
Calories per serving:142; Carbohydrates: 17g; Protein: 6g; Fat: 2g; Fiber: 13g

Instant Pot Vegan Stroganoff

Serves: 2
Preparation Time: 2 minutes
Cooking Time:10 minutes
Ingredients
- 1 ½ cups baby Bella mushrooms, quartered
- 3 cloves of garlic
- 1 cup vegetable stock
- 1 tablespoon sour cream
- Salt and pepper to taste

Instructions
1. Place all ingredients in the Instant Pot.
2. Stir the contents and close the lid.
3. Close the lid and press the Manual button.
4. Adjust the cooking time to 10 minutes.
5. Do quick pressure release.
6. Serve over noodles or rice.

Nutrition information:
Calories per serving: 64; Carbohydrates:11.28 g; Protein: 4.5g; Fat: 1.4g; Fiber: 9.4g

Tomato and Basil Soup

Serves: 8
Preparation Time: 2 minutes
Cooking Time: 10 minutes
Ingredients
- 2 cans whole Roma tomatoes
- ½ cup fresh basil leaves, chopped
- 1 cup vegetable broth
- Salt and pepper to taste
- ¾ cup heavy cream

Instructions
1. Place all ingredients except for the heavy cream in the Instant Pot.
2. Stir the contents and close the lid.
3. Close the lid and press the Manual button.

4. Adjust the cooking time to 8 minutes.
5. Do quick pressure release.
6. Once the lid is open, press the Sauté button and stir in the heavy cream.
7. Allow simmering for 2 minutes.
Nutrition information:
Calories per serving:50; Carbohydrates:2.8 g; Protein:0.86 g; Fat:4.31 g; Fiber: 0.5g

Instant Pot Easy Mushroom Chili

Serves: 3
Preparation Time: 2 minutes
Cooking Time: 10 minutes
Ingredients
- 2 cups diced tomatoes
- 1 15-ounce can baby Bella mushrooms, chopped
- 2 stalks celery
- 1 tablespoon cumin
- 1 teaspoon Mexican spicy seasoning

Instructions
1. Place all ingredients in the Instant Pot.
2. Stir the contents and close the lid.
3. Close the lid and press the Manual button.
4. Adjust the cooking time to 10 minutes.
5. Do quick pressure release.
Nutrition information:
Calories per serving: 70; Carbohydrates:13.15 g; Protein: 4.43g; Fat: 1.3g; Fiber: 6.26g

Crockpot Pumpkin Chili

Serves: 4
Preparation Time: 2 minutes
Cooking Time: 10 minutes
Ingredients
- 3 cups pumpkin, chopped into small pieces
- 3 cups diced tomatoes
- 1 tablespoon chili powder
- 1 tablespoon nutritional yeasts
- 1 can white beans, drained and rinsed
- 1 teaspoon cumin
- Salt and pepper to taste

Instructions
1. Place all ingredients in the Instant Pot.
2. Stir the contents and close the lid.
3. Close the lid and press the Manual button.
4. Adjust the cooking time to 10 minutes.
5. Do quick pressure release.
6. Serve with sour cream and avocado slices if desired.
Nutrition information:
Calories per serving: 120; Carbohydrates: 9.5g; Protein:5.2 g; Fat: 3.2g; Fiber: 7.3g

Vegan Pulled "Pork"

Serves: 6
Preparation Time: 2 minutes
Cooking Time: 25 minutes
Ingredients
- 2 tablespoon olive oil
- ¼ cup chopped onions
- 3 cloves of garlic, minced
- 3 cans green jackfruit, packed in water and drained
- 2 cups barbecue sauce
- 1 teaspoon liquid smoke
- 1 tablespoon Spanish paprika
- 3 tablespoons nutritional yeast
- Salt and pepper

Instructions
1. Press the Sauté button on the Instant Pot and heat oil.
2. Sauté the onions and garlic until fragrant.
3. Add the rest of the ingredients.
4. Close the lid and press the Manual button.
5. Adjust the cooking time to 25 minutes.
6. Do quick pressure release.
Nutrition information:
Calories per serving:207; Carbohydrates: 39g; Protein: 45g; Fat: 8g; Fiber: 32g

Instant Pot Cajun Peanuts

Serves: 6
Preparation Time: 2 minutes
Cooking Time: 10 minutes
Ingredients
- 5 pounds raw peanuts, in shells
- 1 package dry crab boil
- 1 can jalapeno peppers
- 3 tablespoon Cajun seasoning
- 5 cups water

Instructions
1. Place all ingredients in the Instant Pot.
2. Stir the contents and close the lid.
3. Close the lid and press the Manual button.
4. Adjust the cooking time to 4 minutes.
5. Do quick pressure release.
6. Drain the peanuts before serving.
Nutrition information:
Calories per serving:403; Carbohydrates:19 g; Protein: 18.6g; Fat: 37.6g; Fiber: 7g

Indian Coconut Kale Curry

Serves: 4
Preparation Time: 2 minutes
Cooking Time: 4 minutes
Ingredients
- ¼ cup curry powder
- 1 can unsweetened coconut cream
- 1 package dry onion soup mix
- 2 cups kale, rinsed and shredded
- 1 large yellow bell pepper, cut into strips
- 1 cup cilantro for garnish

Instructions
1. Place all ingredients in the Instant Pot.
2. Stir the contents and close the lid.
3. Close the lid and press the Manual button.
4. Adjust the cooking time to 4 minutes.
5. Do quick pressure release.
6. Once the lid is open, garnish with cilantro.
Nutrition information:
Calories per serving: 433; Carbohydrates: 15g; Protein: 10g; Fat: 42.7g; Fiber: 6.7g

Veggie Cheese Soup

Serves: 6
Preparation Time: 2 minutes

Cooking Time: 7 minutes
Ingredients
- 1 package frozen vegetables
- 1 can cream of mushroom soup
- 1 jar cheese sauce
- Salt and pepper to taste
- Mozzarella cheese, shredded

Instructions
1. Place the vegetables in the Instant Pot.
2. Pour the cream of mushroom soup and cheese sauce.
3. Season with salt and pepper. Stir well.
4. Sprinkle mozzarella cheese on top.
5. Close the lid and press the Manual button.
6. Adjust the cooking time to 7 minutes.
7. Do natural pressure release.

Nutrition information:
Calories per serving:196; Carbohydrates: 24.8g; Protein: 9.9g; Fat:6.6 g; Fiber: 5.7g

Instant Pot Zucchini Casserole

Serves: 4
Preparation Time: 2 minutes
Cooking Time: 6 minutes

Ingredients
- 2 zucchinis, sliced
- 1 large onions, chopped
- 4 stalks celery, chopped
- 1 package of your favorite seasoning
- ½ cup vegetable stock
- 4 eggs, beaten
- Salt and pepper

Instructions
1. Place all ingredients in the Instant Pot.
2. Stir the contents and close the lid.
3. Close the lid and press the Manual button.
4. Adjust the cooking time to 4 minutes.
5. Do natural pressure release.

Nutrition information:
Calories per serving:256; Carbohydrates:14.2 g; Protein: 5.7g; Fat: 2.4g; Fiber: 1.8g

Creamy Artichoke, Garlic, And Zucchini

Serves: 12
Preparation Time: 2 minutes
Cooking Time: 10 minutes

Ingredients
- 2 tablespoons coconut oil
- 1 bulb garlic, minced
- 1 large artichoke hearts, cleaned and sliced
- 2 medium zucchinis, sliced
- ½ cup whipping cream
- ½ cup vegetable broth
- Salt and pepper

Instructions
1. Press the Sauté button and heat the oil
2. Sauté the garlic until fragrant.
3. Add the rest of the ingredients.
4. Stir the contents and close the lid.
5. Close the lid and press the Manual button.
6. Adjust the cooking time to 10 minutes.
7. Do quick pressure release.

Nutrition information:
Calories per serving:33; Carbohydrates: 1.79g; Protein:0.57 g; Fat: 2.85g; Fiber: 0.74g

Crockpot Summer Veggies Side Dish

Serves: 6
Preparation Time: 2 minutes
Cooking Time: 7 minutes

Ingredients
- 2 cups okra, sliced
- 1 cup grape tomatoes
- 1 cup mushroom, sliced
- 1 ½ cups onion, sliced
- 2 cups bell pepper, sliced
- 2 ½ cups zucchini, sliced
- 2 tablespoons basil, chopped
- 1 tablespoon thyme, chopped
- ½ cups balsamic vinegar
- ½ cups olive oil
- Salt and pepper

Instructions
1. Place all ingredients in the Instant Pot.
2. Stir the contents and close the lid.
3. Close the lid and press the Manual button.
4. Adjust the cooking time to 7 minutes.
5. Do quick pressure release.

Nutrition information:
Calories per serving:233; Carbohydrates: 7g; Protein: 3g; Fat: 18g; Fiber:4 g

Instant Pot Basic Steamed Vegetables

Serves: 4
Preparation Time: 2 minutes
Cooking Time: 7 minutes

Ingredients
- 2 bell peppers, cut into large slices
- 3 small zucchinis, cut into thick slices
- ½ cup peeled garlic, minced
- 1 tablespoon Italian herb mix
- 2 tablespoon olive oil

Instructions
1. Place all ingredients in a mixing bowl.
2. Season with salt if desired and toss to coat everything.
3. Place a trivet in the Instant Pot and pour 1 cup of water.
4. Place the vegetables on the steamer.
5. Close the lid and press the Steam button.
6. Adjust the cooking time to 7 minutes.
7. Do quick pressure release.

Nutrition information:
Calories per serving:96; Carbohydrates: 8.01g; Protein: 1.75g; Fat: 6.91g; Fiber: 5.3g

Instant Pot French Onion Soup

Serves: 4
Cooking Time: 2 minutes
Preparation Time: 20 minutes

Ingredients
- 6 tablespoon unsalted butter
- 3 pounds onions, chopped
- Salt and pepper to taste
- 3 cups chicken stock
- 1 bay leaf

- 2 sprigs of thyme
- 1 teaspoon fish sauce
- 1 teaspoon apple cider vinegar
- ½ cup dry sherry
- 1 pound cheese, grated
- 1 tablespoon chives for garnish
- 8 slices of bread, toasted

Instructions
1. Press the Sauté button on the Instant Pot.
2. Heat the butter and sauté the onion for 10 minutes until caramelized. Stir constantly.
3. Season with salt and pepper and stir in the rest of the ingredients except for the bread.
4. Stir to combine everything.
5. Place the slices of bread on top.
6. Close the lid and press the Manual button.
7. Adjust the cooking time to 10 minutes.
8. Do natural pressure release.

Nutrition information:
Calories per serving: 749; Carbohydrates:70.1g; Protein: 30.01g; Fat:45.18g; Fiber: 5.3g

Steamed Vegetables Side Dish

Serves: 6
Preparation Time: 2 minutes
Cooking Time:10 minutes

Ingredients
- 2 bell peppers, sliced
- 2 large zucchinis, sliced
- ½ cup peeled garlic cloves
- Salt and pepper to taste
- 1 teaspoon Italian seasoning
- 2 tablespoons olive oil
- ¼ cup parmesan cheese, grated

Instructions
1. Place a trivet or steamer in the Instant Pot and pour a cup of water.
2. In a baking dish that will fit inside the Instant Pot, mix the pepper, zucchini, and garlic. Season with salt, pepper, and Italian seasoning.
3. Pour in olive oil and toss to combine.
4. Add the parmesan cheese on top.
5. Place on top of the steamer basket.
6. Close the lid and press the Steam button.
7. Adjust the cooking time to 10 minutes.
8. Do quick pressure release.

Nutrition information:
Calories per serving: 127; Carbohydrates:8.6 g; Protein: 2g; Fat: 15.3g; Fiber: 6.1g

Vegan Miso Risotto

Serves: 6
Cooking Time: 2 minutes
Preparation Time: 10 minutes

Ingredients
- 6 tablespoon olive oil
- 1 medium onion, chopped finely
- 3 cloves garlic, chopped
- 2 cups Arborio or risotto rice
- 2 teaspoon soy sauce
- ¾ cup dry sake
- ¼ cup miso paste
- ½ teaspoon juice of 1 lemon
- 4 cups vegetable stock
- Salt to taste
- Chives for garnish

Instructions
1. Press the Sauté button on the Instant Pot.
2. Heat the oil and sauté the onion and garlic until fragrant.
3. Stir in the Arborio rice and add the rest of the ingredients except for the chives.
4. Close the lid and press the Rice button.
5. Adjust the cooking time to 6 minutes
6. Do natural pressure release.
7. Garnish with chopped chives.

Nutrition information:
Calories per serving: 936; Carbohydrates: 19.4g; Protein: 4.27g; Fat: 89g; Fiber: 6.1g

Farro And Cherry Salad

Serves: 5
Cooking Time:5 minutes
Preparation Time: 40 minutes

Ingredients
- 1 cup raw grain farro
- 1 tablespoon apple cider vinegar
- 1 teaspoon lemon juice
- ¼ teaspoon salt
- 1 tablespoon olive oil
- ¼ cup chives, minced
- ¼ cup dried cherries, chopped
- 8 mint leaves, minced
- 2 cups fresh cherries, pitted and halved

Instructions
1. Place the faro in the Instant Pot and add 3 cups of water.
2. Close the lid and press the Rice button.
3. Adjust the cooking time to 40 minutes.
4. Do natural pressure release.
5. Allow the farro grains cool for a few minutes.
6. Place in a salad bowl and combine the remaining ingredients.
7. Toss to mix well.

Nutrition information:
Calories per serving:209; Carbohydrates:35.53g; Protein: 6.12g; Fat:5.53g; Fiber: 3.8g

Savory Mashed Sweet Potatoes

Serves: 8
Cooking Time: 2 minutes
Preparation Time: 15 minutes

Ingredients
- 1 pound sweet potatoes, peeled and cut into cubes
- 2 cloves of garlic
- Salt and pepper to taste
- ½ teaspoon dried parsley
- ¼ teaspoon dried thyme
- ¼ teaspoon dried rosemary
- ¼ teaspoon dried sage
- 2 tablespoons butter
- ¼ cup milk
- ½ cup parmesan, grated

Instructions
1. Place a trivet or steamer basket in the pressure cooker. Add a cup of water.

2. Place the sweet potatoes and garlic on top of the steamer basket.
3. Close the lid and press the Steam button.
4. Adjust the cooking time to 15 minutes.
5. Do quick pressure release once the pressure cooker is done.
6. Mash the potatoes with the rest of the ingredients.
7. Serve warm.
Nutrition information:
Calories per serving: 354; Carbohydrates: 35.39g; Protein: 4.1g; Fat: 21.74g; Fiber: 5.1g

Sun-Dried Tomato Polenta

Serves: 8
Cooking Time: 2 minutes
Preparation Time: 10 minutes
Ingredients
- 2 tablespoons olive oil
- 2 cloves of garlic, minced
- ½ cup onion, chopped
- 4 cups vegetable stock
- 1/3 cup sun-dried tomatoes, finely chopped
- 1 bay leaf
- 1 teaspoon salt
- 2 tablespoons parsley, chopped
- 2 teaspoons oregano, chopped
- 3 tablespoons basil, chopped
- 1 teaspoon rosemary, chopped
- 1 cup polenta

Instructions
1. Press the Sauté button on the Instant Pot and add the oil.
2. Sauté the garlic and onions for 3 minutes until fragrant.
3. Add the stock, sun-dried tomatoes, bay leaf, salt, parsley, oregano, basil, and rosemary. Stir to combine.
4. Sprinkle polenta on top but do not stir.
5. Close the lid and adjust the cooking time to 5 minutes.
6. Do natural pressure release.
Nutrition information:
Calories per serving: 69; Carbohydrates: 8.48g; Protein: 1.07g; Fat: 3.61g; Fiber: 0.9g

Spicy Thai Quinoa Salad

Serves: 8
Cooking Time: 30 minutes
Preparation Time: 30 minutes
Ingredients
- 1 cup quinoa
- 1 ½ cups water
- ½ teaspoon salt
- 1 carrot, shredded
- 6 green onions, chopped
- 1 cucumber, chopped
- 1 cup edamame
- 2 cups red cabbage, shredded
- ¼ cup lime juice
- 1 tablespoon soy sauce
- 1 tablespoon vegetable oil
- 2 tablespoons sugar
- 1 tablespoon sesame oil
- 1 tablespoon ginger, grated
- ½ cup peanuts, toasted and chopped
- A pinch of red pepper flakes
- 2 tablespoons basil, chopped
- ¼ cup cilantro, chopped

Instructions
1. Place the quinoa, water, and salt in the Instant Pot.
2. Close the lid and press the Multigrain button.
3. Adjust the cooking time to 30 minutes. Once done cooking, do quick pressure release.
4. Transfer the quinoa to a bowl and let it cool for at least 30 minutes.
5. Once cooled, mix quinoa with carrots, onions, cucumber, edamame, and cabbage. Mix well to combine. Set aside.
6. In another mixing bowl, mix together the lime juice, soy sauce, vegetable oil, sugar, sesame oil, ginger, peanuts, red pepper flakes, basil, and cilantro.
7. Pour the sauce over the quinoa salad.
Nutrition information:
Calories per serving: 271; Carbohydrates: 31.78g; Protein: 11.16g; Fat:12.55g; Fiber: 5.4g

Rice Pilaf with Vegetables

Serves: 10
Cooking Time: 2 minutes
Preparation Time: 5 minutes
Ingredients
- 1 tablespoon butter
- 1 medium onion, chopped
- 1 carrot, chopped
- 1 celery stalk, chopped
- 2 cups long grain white rice
- 1 can chicken broth
- ½ teaspoon salt
- 1 ¼ cup water
- 1 cup peas
- ½ cup almonds, slivered
- 2 tablespoons parsley, chopped

Instructions
1. Press the Sauté button on the Instant Pot and melt the butter.
2. Sauté the onions, carrots, and celery for 3 minutes or until the vegetables are translucent.
3. Stir in the rice and stir constantly for 2 minutes.
4. Add the rest of the ingredients.
5. Close the lid and press the Rice button.
6. Adjust the cooking time to 6 minutes.
7. Do natural pressure release.
8. Open the lid and press the Sauté button.
Nutrition information:
Calories per serving:163; Carbohydrates:31.56 g; Protein:4.32g; Fat: 1.78g; Fiber: 0.9g

Grains and Kale Salad

Serves: 12
Cooking Time: 30 minutes
Preparation Time: 3 minutes
Ingredients
- 1 package of harvest grains of your choice
- 1 teaspoon salt
- 2 ½ cups water
- 1/3 cup red onion, diced
- 3 cups kale leaves, torn

- 4 tablespoon lemon juice
- 1/3 cup extra-virgin olive oil
- Zest of 1 lemon
- Salt and pepper to taste
- ¼ cup feta cheese, crumbled

Instructions
1. Place the harvest grains, salt, and water in the Instant Pot.
2. Close the lid and press the Rice button.
3. Adjust the cooking time to 3 minutes.
4. Do natural pressure release and allow the grains to cool down.
5. Place the grains in a large bowl.
6. Mix in the grains and the rest of the ingredients. Mix well to combine everything.
7. Serve warm.

Nutrition information:
Calories per serving: 55; Carbohydrates: 4.95g; Protein: 0.87g; Fat: 3.65g; Fiber: 0.4g

Pressure Cooker Mashed Potatoes

Serves: 8
Cooking Time: 2 minutes
Preparation Time: 5 minutes

Ingredients
- 2 pounds potatoes, peeled and quartered
- 2/3 cup milk
- 1 cup water
- 4 tablespoons butter
- Salt and pepper to taste

Instructions
1. Place a steamer basket in the Instant Pot. Pour a cup of water.
2. Place the potatoes on top of the steamer.
3. Close the lid and press the Steam button.
4. Adjust the cooking time to 30 minutes.
5. Do natural pressure release.
6. Transfer the potatoes to a bowl and mash together with the other ingredients.
7. Serve warm.

Nutrition information:
Calories per serving: 153; Carbohydrates:21.32g; Protein: 3.11g; Fat: 6.54g; Fiber: 2.6g

Aromatic Rosemary Garlic Potatoes

Serves: 4
Cooking Time: 2 minutes
Preparation Time: 30 minutes

Ingredients
- 1 pound potatoes, peeled and sliced thinly
- 2 garlic cloves
- ½ teaspoon salt
- 1 tablespoon olive oil
- 2 sprigs of rosemary

Instructions
1. Place a trivet or steamer basket in the Instant Pot and pour in a cup of water.
2. In a baking dish that can fit inside the Instant Pot, combine all ingredients and toss to coat everything.
3. Cover the baking dish with aluminum foil and place on the steamer basket.
4. Close the lid and press the Steam button.
5. Adjust the cooking time to 30 minutes
6. Do quick pressure release.

Nutrition information:
Calories per serving: 119; Carbohydrates: 20.31g; Protein: 2.39g; Fat: 3.48g; Fiber: 2.5g

Simple Green Beans Salad

Serves: 8
Cooking Time: 2 minutes
Preparation Time: 6 minutes

Ingredients
- 1 ounce dried porcini mushrooms, soaked overnight and rinsed
- 2 pounds potatoes, sliced to 1-inch thick
- 2 pounds green beans, trimmed and cleaned
- 1 cup boiling water
- Salt and pepper
- 1 tablespoon olive oil
- 1 tablespoon balsamic vinegar

Instructions
1. Place the mushrooms, potatoes, and beans in the Instant Pot.
2. Pour enough water to boil.
3. Close the lid and press the Manual button.
4. Adjust the cooking time to 6 minutes.
5. Do quick pressure release.
6. Take the vegetables out and drain the water.
7. Place the veggies to cool in a salad bowl
8. Toss in salt, pepper, olive oil, and balsamic vinegar.
9. Toss to coat.

Nutrition information:
Calories per serving: 181; Carbohydrates: 32.4g; Protein: 8.1g; Fat: 3.2g; Fiber: 6.5g

Creamy Cheese Au Gratin

Serves: 8
Cooking Time: 10 minutes
Preparation Time: 20 minutes

Ingredients
- 2 tablespoons butter
- ½ cup onion, chopped
- 1 cup chicken broth
- 6 medium potatoes, sliced
- Salt and pepper to taste
- ½ cup sour cream
- 1 cup Monterey jack cheese, shredded
- 3 tablespoons butter, solid

Instructions
1. Press the Sauté button on the Instant Pot and melt the butter
2. Sauté the onion until fragrant.
3. Add the chicken broth and tomatoes. Season with salt and pepper.
4. Stir in the sour cream and cheese.
5. Close the lid and adjust the cooking time to 20 minutes.
6. Do natural pressure release.
7. Once the lid is open, add the butter.
8. Allow it to melt on top of the cheese.

Nutrition information:
Calories per serving: 376; Carbohydrates: 52.99g; Protein: 10.99g; Fat: 14.2g; Fiber: 6.4g

Sweet Sticky Carrots

Serves: 8
Cooking Time: 2 minutes
Preparation Time: 10 minutes
Ingredients
- 2 pounds carrots, peeled and sliced thickly
- ¼ cup raisins
- 1 tablespoon butter, melted
- 1 tablespoon maple syrup
- Pepper to taste

Instructions
1. Place the carrots and raisins in the Instant Pot.
2. Add a cup of water and close the lid.
3. Press the Steam button and adjust the cooking time to 6 minutes.
4. Do natural pressure release to open the lid.
5. Drain the carrots and raisins to remove excess water.
6. Meanwhile, press the Sauté button on the Instant Pot and heat the butter. Stir in the maple syrup and add the carrots and raisins back to the pressure cooker. Add pepper to taste.
7. Allow simmering for 2 minutes.

Nutrition information:
Calories per serving: 63; Carbohydrates:11.55g; Protein: 0.99g; Fat:1.83g; Fiber: 3.5g

Brussels Sprouts With Pine Nuts and Pomegranate Seeds

Serves: 6
Cooking Time: 2 minutes
Preparation Time: 5 minutes
Ingredients
- 1 pound Brussels sprouts, trimmed and cleaned
- ¼ cup pine nuts, toasted
- 1 pomegranate, seeds saved
- 1 tablespoon olive oil
- Salt and pepper

Instructions
1. Place a trivet or steamer basket inside the pressure cooker and add a cup of water
2. Place the Brussels sprouts on the steamer and close the lid.
3. Press the Steam button and cook on preset cooking time.
4. Do natural pressure release.
5. Transfer the Brussels sprouts in a salad bowl.
6. Add the rest of the ingredients to the Brussels sprouts.
7. Toss to mix the ingredients.

Nutrition information:
Calories per serving: 132; Carbohydrates:17.04g; Protein: 4.22g; Fat: 6.9g; Fiber: 5.1g

Smoking Hot Pickled Green Chilies

Serves: 8
Cooking Time: 2 minutes
Preparation Time: 4 minutes
Ingredients
- 1 pound green chilies or jalapeno peppers, sliced
- 1 teaspoon canning salt
- ¼ teaspoon garlic powder
- 1 ½ cups apple cider vinegar
- 1 ½ teaspoon sugar

Instructions
1. Place all ingredients in the Instant Pot.
2. Stir the contents and close the lid.
3. Close the lid and press the Manual button.
4. Adjust the cooking time to 4 minutes.
5. Do quick pressure release.

Nutrition information:
Calories per serving: 3.1; Carbohydrates: 0.6g; Protein: 0.1g; Fat: 0g; Fiber: 0.2g

Simple Pressure Cooker Chickpea Hummus

Serves: 8
Cooking Time: 2 minutes
Preparation Time: 40minutes
Ingredients
- 1 cup dried chickpeas, soaked overnight
- 4 cloves of garlic
- 1 bay leaf
- 2 tablespoon tahini
- 1 juice of lemon
- ¼ teaspoon cumin
- ½ teaspoon salt
- A dash of paprika
- ½ teaspoon parsley
- A dash of extra virgin olive oil

Instructions
1. Place the chickpeas in the Instant Pot and add 6 cups of water.
2. Close the lid of the pressure cooker and press the Beans/Chili button and adjust the cooking time for 40 minutes.
3. Do natural pressure release.
4. Transfer the chickpeas to a food processor and add the garlic, tahini, lemon, cumin, and salt.
5. Pulse until smooth.
6. Transfer to a bowl and garnish with paprika, parsley and olive oil.

Nutrition information:
Calories per serving: 109.1; Carbohydrates: 0.2g; Protein: 4.1g; Fat: 3.8g; Fiber: 3.3g

Simple Eggplant Spread

Serves: 6
Cooking Time: 5 minutes
Preparation Time: 5 minutes
Ingredients
- 4 tablespoon olive oil
- 2 pounds eggplant, sliced
- 4 garlic cloves
- 1 teaspoon salt
- 1 cup water
- 1 lemon, juiced
- 1 tablespoon tahini
- ¼ cup black olives, pitted and sliced
- A few sprigs of thyme
- A dash of extra virgin oil

Instructions
1. Press the Sauté button on the pressure cooker.
2. Heat the oil and add the sliced eggplants. Fry the eggplants for 3 minutes on each side.
3. Stir in the garlic and sauté until fragrant. Season with salt.

4. Add a cup of water and close the lid.
5. Press the Manual button and adjust the cooking time to 6 minutes.
6. Do natural pressure release and take the eggplants out and transfer to a food processor.
7. Add salt, lemon juice, and tahini.
8. Pulse until smooth.
9. Place in a bowl and garnish with olives, thyme and a dash of extra virgin olive oil.
Nutrition information:
Calories per serving: 155; Carbohydrates: 16.8g; Protein: 2g; Fat:11.7g; Fiber: 4.5g

Steamed Savory Artichokes

Serves: 4
Cooking Time: 2 minutes
Preparation Time: 10 minutes
Ingredients
- 2 artichokes, trimmed and halved
- 1 lemon, sliced in half
- 2 tablespoons mayonnaise
- 1 teaspoon Dijon mustard
- A pinch of paprika

Instructions
1. Place a steamer basket in the Instant Pot and pour a cup of water
2. Place the artichokes on top of the steamer basket. Spritz the artichokes with lemon juice.
3. Close the lid and press the Steam button.
4. Adjust the cooking time to 10 minutes.
5. Do natural pressure release.
6. Meanwhile, mix together mayonnaise, mustard, and paprika.
7. Serve artichokes with the sauce
Nutrition information:
Calories per serving:77.5; Carbohydrates: 0g; Protein:2g; Fat: 5g; Fiber: 3.5g

Creamy Bean and Artichoke Dip

Serves: 8
Cooking Time: 15 minutes
Preparation Time: 50 minutes
Ingredients
- ½ cup dry cannellini beans, soaked overnight
- 8 medium-sized artichokes, cleaned and trimmed
- 1 cup water
- ½ lemon, juiced
- 2 cloves of garlic, minced
- ¾ cup plain non-fat yogurt
- 1 teaspoon salt
- ¼ teaspoon pepper
- ¾ cup grated Parmigiano cheese

Instructions
1. Place the beans, artichokes, and water in the Instant Pot.
2. Close the lid and press the Bean/Chili button.
3. Adjust the cooking time to 50 minutes.
4. Do quick pressure release.
5. Drain the beans and allow to remove excess water.
6. In a food processor, place the beans and artichokes.
7. Season with lemon juice, garlic, yogurt, salt, and pepper.
8. Pulse until smooth.
9. Add the grated Parmigiano cheese.
Nutrition information:
Calories per serving: 134; Carbohydrates: 20.95g; Protein: 9.36g; Fat:3.27g; Fiber: 9g

Instant Pot Steamed Artichoke

Serves: 8
Cooking Time: 5 minutes
Preparation Time: 5 minutes
Ingredients:
- 2 cups water
- 2 lemons, one sliced and one juiced
- 6 artichokes, cleaned and trimmed
- 1 tablespoon peppercorns
- 3 cloves of garlic, minced
- 2 cups olive oil

Instructions
1. Pour the water and juice from one lemon in the pressure cooker.
2. Place the artichokes, peppercorns, garlic and olive oil in the pressure cooker
3. Close the lid and press the Manual button.
4. Adjust the cooking time to 5 minutes.
5. Do quick pressure release.
Nutrition information:
Calories per serving: 548; Carbohydrates:14.03g; Protein: 4.11g; Fat: 45.55g; Fiber: 6.6g

Asian Sesame Noodles

Serves: 6
Cooking Time: 6 minutes
Preparation Time: 5 minutes
Ingredients
- 16 ounces Chinese egg noodles
- 3 1/5 cups of water
- ½ cup soy sauce
- 6 tablespoon sesame oil
- 8 cloves of garlic, minced
- 4 tablespoons sugar
- 4 tablespoon rice vinegar
- 8 tablespoon canola oil
- 1 teaspoon hot chili oil
- 8 scallions, sliced thinly

Instructions
1. Pour water into the Instant Pot and add the noodles.
2. Close the lid and press the Manual button.
3. Adjust cooking time to 6 minutes.
4. Once the timer beeps off, do quick pressure release.
5. Drain the noodles and allow to cool.
6. Meanwhile, mix the soy sauce, sesame oil, garlic, sugar, rice vinegar, canola oil, and chili oil in a mixing bowl.
7. Pour over the sauce and mix.
8. Stir in the scallions.
Nutrition information:
Calories per serving:522; Carbohydrates: 14.58g; Protein: 11.82g; Fat: 46.58g; Fiber:1g

Simple Rice Salad

Serves: 5
Cooking Time: 30 minutes
Preparation Time: 8 minutes

Ingredients
- 2 cups Arborio rice
- 4 cups water
- A pinch of salt
- A dash of olive oil
- 2 fresh tomatoes, chopped
- 3 hard-boiled eggs, chopped
- 1 cup black olives, chopped
- 1 bunch basil, chopped
- 4 ounces of cooked ham, diced
- 1 mozzarella ball, sliced
- 3 tablespoon pickled capers
- A dash of olive oil

Instructions
1. Place the rice, water, salt and olive oil inside the Instant Pot.
2. Close the lid and press the Rice button. Cook for 8 minutes.
3. Do natural pressure release.
4. Transfer the rice to a salad bowl and allow to cool for at least 30 minutes.
5. Once cooled, toss the remaining ingredients.
6. Toss to combine all ingredients.

Nutrition information:
Calories per serving: 256; Carbohydrates: 27.32g; Protein: 14.8g; Fat: 16.5g; Fiber: 11.3g

Spicy Brown Rice Salad with Black Beans

Serves: 8
Cooking Time: 30 minutes
Preparation Time: 10 minutes

Ingredients
- 1 cup brown rice
- ¼ teaspoon salt
- 1 ½ cups water
- 12 grape tomatoes, halved
- 1 can black beans, drained and rinsed
- ¼ cup minced cilantro
- 1 avocado, diced
- 3 tablespoon lime juice
- 2 teaspoon Tabasco sauce
- 1 teaspoon honey
- 2 garlic cloves
- 1/8 teaspoon salt
- 3 tablespoon olive oil

Instructions
1. Place the rice, salt, and water in the Instant Pot.
2. Close the lid and press the Rice button.
3. Adjust the cooking time to 10 minutes.
4. Do natural pressure release.
5. Place rice in a bowl. Let the rice cool for at least 30 minutes.
6. Once the rice has cooled off, add tomatoes, black beans, cilantro, and avocado. Mix well to combine. Set aside.
7. Prepare the dressing by mixing together the remaining ingredients.
8. Pour the dressing over the rice salad.

Nutrition information:
Calories per serving: 130; Carbohydrates: 10.74g; Protein: 2.47g; Fat: 9.27g; Fiber: 4.4g

Dessert Recipes

Sweet Apple Pudding

Serves: 6
Preparation Time: 5 minutes
Cooking Time: 15 minutes

Ingredients
- ½ cup coconut sugar
- 2 cups milk
- ¼ teaspoon allspice
- ¼ teaspoon nutmeg, ground
- 2 teaspoons cinnamon
- 2 tablespoon lemon juice
- 6 medium apples, deseeded and chopped
- ½ cup raw honey
- 2 teaspoons vanilla
- 1 teaspoon sea salt

Instructions
1. Place all ingredients in the Instant Pot.
2. Give a good stir.
3. Close the lid and press the Manual button.
4. Adjust the cooking time to 10 minutes.
5. Do natural pressure release.

Nutrition information:
Calories per serving:271; Carbohydrates:61.9 g; Protein: 3.1g; Fat: 3.4g; Fiber: 4.9g

Instant Pot "Baked" Apples

Serves: 6
Preparation Time: 5 minutes
Cooking Time: 10 minutes

Ingredients
- 6 apples, cored
- ½ cup brown sugar
- 1 cup red wine
- ¼ cup raisins
- 1 teaspoon cinnamon powder

Instructions
1. Place the apples on the bottom of the pressure cooker.
2. Add the rest of the ingredients on top.
3. Do not stir the mixture
4. Close the lid and press the Manual button.
5. Adjust the cooking time to 10 minutes.
6. Do natural pressure release.
7. Serve with your favorite ice cream.

Nutrition information:
Calories per serving: 188.7; Carbohydrates: 41.9g; Protein: 0.6g; Fat: 0.3g; Fiber: 3.8g

Instant Pot Oreo Cheesecake

Serves: 6
Preparation Time: 20 minutes
Cooking Time: 10 minutes

Ingredients
- 12 Oreo cookies, crushed
- 2 tablespoons butter, melted
- 16 ounces cream cheese
- ½ cup granulated sugar
- 2 large eggs
- 1 tablespoon all-purpose flour
- ¼ cup heavy cream
- 2 teaspoon vanilla extract

- 8 whole Oreo cookies, chopped

Instructions
1. Place a steamer rack in the Instant Pot and pour a cup of water.
2. Get a springform pan that will fit in the Instant Pot. Wrap a spring-form pan in foil and spray the inside of the pan with oil. Set aside.
3. In a mixing bowl, mix the crushed Oreo cookies and melted butter. Press the crumbs on the bottom of the pan. Refrigerate the pan.
4. In a bowl, beat the cream cheese until smooth. Add the sugar and eggs slowly until well combined. Add in flour, cream, and vanilla. Fold in the chopped Oreo cookies.
5. Pour the batter into the prepared crust.
6. Place an aluminum foil on top of the springform pan.
7. Place the pan inside the pressure cooker and close the lid.
8. Press the Steam button and adjust the cooking time to 10 minutes.
9. Do natural pressure release.
10. Allow to cool before serving.

Nutrition information:
Calories per serving: 597; Carbohydrates: 42.34g; Protein: 9.71g; Fat: 44.2g; Fiber: 1.2g

Asian Coconut Rice Pudding

Serves: 8
Preparation Time: 2 minutes
Cooking Time: 10 minutes

Ingredients
- 1 ½ cups sticky rice
- ¾ cup sugar
- ½ teaspoon salt
- 3 cups coconut milk
- 1 stalk pandan leaf

Instructions
1. Put everything in the Instant Pot.
2. Give a good stir.
3. Close the lid and press the Rice button.
4. Adjust the cooking time to 10 minutes.
5. Do natural pressure release.
6. Discard the pandan leaf.

Nutrition information:
Calories per serving: 193; Carbohydrates: 29.14g; Protein: 3.81g; Fat: 17.8g Fiber: 4.6g

Instant Pot Crème Brule

Serves: 6
Preparation Time: 6 minutes
Cooking Time: 20 minutes

Ingredients
- 8 egg yolks
- 1/3 cup granulated sugar
- A pinch of salt
- 1 ½ teaspoon vanilla
- 2 cups of heavy cream
- 6 tablespoon fine sugar

Instructions
1. Place a steamer rack in the Instant Pot and pour a cup of water.
2. In a mixing bowl, combine the egg yolks, granulated sugar, and salt.
3. Pour in vanilla and cream and whisk until well combined.
4. Strain the mixture to remove any lumps and pour into ramekin cups.
5. Cover the ramekin cups with aluminum foil.
6. Place on top of the steamer rack.
7. Press the Steam button and adjust the cooking time to 6 minutes.
8. Do natural pressure release.
9. Remove and sprinkle sugar over the custard.

Nutrition information:
Calories per serving: 267; Carbohydrates: 15.53g; Protein: 4.42g; Fat: 20.82g; Fiber: 0g

Pumpkin and Rice Pudding

Serves: 6
Preparation Time: 10 minutes
Cooking Time: 35 minutes

Ingredients
- 1 cup short grain rice
- 3 cups milk
- ½ cup water
- ½ cups pitted dates, chopped
- 1/8 teaspoon salt
- 1 stick cinnamon stick
- 1 cup pumpkin puree
- 1 teaspoon pumpkin spice mix
- ½ cup maple syrup
- 1 teaspoon vanilla extract

Instructions
1. Soak rice with water and let it rest for at least 10 minutes.
2. Without the lid on, press the Sauté button on the Instant Pot and add milk and water. Add the rice. Bring to a boil and add rice, dates, and cinnamon. Season with salt.
3. Lock the lid and press the Rice button.
4. Adjust the cooking time to 20 minutes.
5. Do natural pressure release to open the lid.
6. Once the lid is open, press the Sauté button and add the pumpkin puree, spice mix, maple syrup and vanilla extract.
7. Allow simmering for 5 minutes
8. Remove the cinnamon stick before serving.

Nutrition information:
Calories per serving: 412; Carbohydrates: 62.23g; Protein: 12.2g; Fat: 13.87g; Fiber: 3.3g

Steamed Cranberry Pudding

Serves: 6
Preparation Time: 15 minutes
Cooking Time: 25 minutes

Ingredients
- 4 eggs, beaten
- ½ cup granulated sugar
- cups milk
- 1 teaspoon vanilla
- 3 cups bread cubes
- 1/3 cup dried cranberries
- 1/3 cup pecans, chopped

Instructions

1. Place a trivet or steamer rack in the pressure cooker. Pour a cup of water.
2. Grease a ramekin dish that will fit inside the pressure cooker.
3. In a mixing bowl, combine the eggs, sugar, and milk using a whisk.
4. Stir in the vanilla.
5. Arrange the bread cubes and cranberries in the ramekin dish.
6. Pour the custard mixture. Place tin foil on top of the dish.
7. Place the dish on the steamer rack.
8. Close the lid in place and press the Steam button. Adjust the cooking time to 25 minutes.
9. Do natural pressure release.
10. Top with pecans and refrigerate for at least 8 hours to harden.

Nutrition information:
Calories per serving: 237; Carbohydrates: 22.31g; Protein: 9.31g; Fat:12.28g; Fiber: 1g

Sweet Coconut Tapioca

Serves: 8
Preparation Time: 10 minutes
Cooking Time: 5 minutes

Ingredients
- 1 cup pearl tapioca, rinsed
- 5 cups coconut milk
- 16-inch lemongrass, smashed
- 2 teaspoons ginger, grated
- 1 cup sugar
- 4 egg yolks
- ½ teaspoon salt
- 1 cup cashew nuts, toasted

Instructions
1. Place tapioca pearls and coconut milk in the Instant Pot.
2. Stir in lemongrass and ginger.
3. Close the lid and press the Rice button.
4. Adjust the cooking time to 6 minutes.
5. Do natural pressure release.
6. Meanwhile, mix the sugar, egg yolks and salt in a mixing bowl.
7. Once the lid is open, press the Sauté button and pour the egg mixture.
8. Allow simmering until the mixture thickens.
9. Top with toasted cashew nuts.

Nutrition information:
Calories per serving: 692; Carbohydrates: 55.95g; Protein: 9.02g; Fat: 51.75g; Fiber: 4.4g

Steamed Key Lime Pie

Serves: 8
Preparation Time: 15 minutes
Cooking Time: 15 minutes

Ingredients
- ¾ cup graham cracker crumbs
- 3 tablespoons butter, melted
- 1 tablespoon sugar
- 1 can condensed milk
- 4 large egg yolks
- ½ cup key lime juice
- 1/3 cup sour cream
- 2 tablespoon key lime zest

Instructions
1. Place a trivet or steamer rack in the Instant Pot and pour a cup of water.
2. Coat a springform pan that will fit in the pressure cooker with cooking spray.
3. In a bowl, mix together the graham crackers, butter, and sugar. Press evenly on the bottom of the pan to form the crust. Place in the fridge to set.
4. In another bowl, beat the egg yolks until light yellow.
5. Stir in the condensed milk. Beat in the lime juice and beat until smooth. Stir the sour cream and lime zest.
6. Pour the batter into the springform pan and cover the top with aluminum foil.
7. Place on the steamer rack and close the lid.
8. Press the Steam button and adjust the cooking time to 15 minutes.
9. Do natural pressure release.
10. Allow to cool in the fridge before serving.

Nutrition information:
Calories per serving: 93; Carbohydrates: 4.67g; Protein: 1.9g; Fat: 7.74g; Fiber: 0.1g

Dulce De Leche

Serves: 4
Preparation Time: 10 minutes
Cooking Time: 30 minutes

Ingredients
- 1 can sweetened condensed milk

Instructions
1. Place a steamer basket in the Instant Pot and add 8 cups of water.
2. Pour the condensed milk into a 16-ounce canning jar.
3. Place the jar with the condensed milk on the steamer rack.
4. Place the jar with condensed milk on the steamer rack.
5. Close the lid and press the Steam button.
6. Adjust the cooking time to 30 minutes.
7. Do natural pressure release.

Nutrition information:
Calories per serving: 525; Carbohydrates: 84.26g; Protein: 8.16g; Fat: 17.8g; Fiber: 2.2g

Fast Pressure Cooker Hazelnut Flan

Serves: 4
Preparation Time: 15 minutes
Cooking Time: 50 minutes

Ingredients
- 1 1/4 cups granulated sugar
- ¼ cup water
- 3 eggs
- 2 egg yolks
- A pinch of salt
- 2 cups milk
- ½ cup whipping cream
- 1 teaspoon vanilla extract
- 2 tablespoon hazelnut syrup

Instructions

1. Prepare the caramel base by heating the ¾ cup sugar and ¼ cup water. Bring to a boil and place on ramekins before it hardens. Set aside.
2. Place a trivet or steamer basket in the pressure cooker and a cup of water.
3. In a mixing bowl, beat the eggs, yolks and the remaining cup of sugar. Add a pinch of salt.
4. Heat milk in a saucepan over medium heat until it bubbles. Add milk to eggs to temper the eggs.
5. Stir in the cream, vanilla and Hazelnut syrup.
6. Pour mixture into ramekins and cover with tin foil.
7. Place in the steamer basket and close the lid.
8. Press the Steam button and adjust the cooking time to 50 minutes.
9. Do natural pressure release.
Nutrition information:
Calories per serving: 325; Carbohydrates:35.12g; Protein: 12.16g; Fat: 15.16g; Fiber: 0g

Steamed Carrot Pudding Cake

Serves: 8
Preparation Time: 20 minutes
Cooking Time: 50 minutes
Ingredients
- 1 cup brown sugar
- ¼ cup molasses
- 2 eggs
- ½ cup flour
- ½ teaspoon cinnamon
- ½ teaspoon allspice
- ½ teaspoon nutmeg
- ½ teaspoon baking soda
- ¼ teaspoon salt
- 2/3 cup shortening, frozen and grated
- ½ cup carrots, grated
- ½ cup raisins
- 1 cup breadcrumbs
- ½ cup pecans, chopped
- 4 tablespoons butter
- ¼ cup cream
- 2 tablespoons rum
- ¼ teaspoon cinnamon, ground

Instructions
1. Place a steamer rack in the Instant Pot and add a cup of water.
2. In a mixing bowl, whisk ½ cup of brown sugar, molasses, and eggs.
3. Pour in the flour and the spices, baking soda, salt, shortening, carrots, bread crumbs, and pecans.
4. Pour the batter into a baking dish that will fit the pressure cooker. Cover with aluminum foil and place on the steamer.
5. Close the lid and press the Steam button.
6. Adjust the cooking time to 50 minutes.
7. Prepare the rum sauce by mixing in a saucepan the remaining brown sugar, butter, cream, rum, and cinnamon. Heat over low flame until reduced.
8. Once the pressure cooker beeps, do natural pressure release.
9. Pour over the rum sauce on top.
10. Allow to cool before serving.
Nutrition information:
Calories per serving:428; Carbohydrates:31.92g; Protein: 4.27g; Fat: 31.55g; Fiber: 1.3g

Coconut Pina Colada Pudding

Serves: 8
Preparation Time: 10 minutes
Cooking Time: 11 minutes
Ingredients
- 1 cup Arborio rice
- 1 ½ cups water
- 1 tablespoon coconut oil
- ¼ teaspoon salt
- 1 can coconut milk
- 2 eggs
- ½ cup milk
- ½ teaspoon vanilla extract
- 1 can pineapple tidbits, drained

Instructions
1. Mix the rice, water, and oil in the Instant Pot. Season with salt.
2. Close the lid and press the Rice button. Adjust the cooking time to 6 minutes.
3. Do natural pressure release to open the lid.
4. Meanwhile, beat the eggs, milk, and vanilla. Pour over the sieve to remove any lumps.
5. Once the lid is open, press the Sauté and pour over the coconut milk and sugar. Stir to mix everything.
6. Add the egg mixture until it thickens.
7. Stir in the pineapples last.
Nutrition information:
Calories per serving: 152; Carbohydrates: 20.31g; Protein: 5.04g; Fat:7.71g; Fiber: 3.3g

Pumpkin and Chocolate Bundt Cake

Serves: 8
Preparation Time: 15 minutes
Cooking Time: 50 minutes
Ingredients
- 1 ½ cups all-purpose flour
- ½ teaspoon pumpkin pie spice
- 1 teaspoon ground cinnamon
- ¼ teaspoon salt
- ½ teaspoon baking soda
- ½ teaspoon baking powder
- ½ cup butter softened
- 1 cup granulated sugar
- 2 eggs
- 1 cup pumpkin puree
- ¾ cup mini chocolate chips

Instructions
1. Place a trivet or steamer rack in the Instant Pot and a cup of water.
2. In a mixing bowl, mix the flour, pumpkin pie spice, cinnamon, salt, baking soda and baking powder.
3. In another bowl, beat in the rest of the ingredients until fluffy.
4. Mix the dry ingredients and wet ingredients.
5. Pour the batter into greased Bundt pan that will fit inside the Instant Pot. Cover with aluminum foil.
6. Place on top of the steamer and close the lid.
7. Press the Steam button and adjust the cooking time to 50 minutes.
8. Do natural pressure release.
Nutrition information:
Calories per serving: 354; Carbohydrates: 33.27g; Protein: 9.2g; Fat: 21.4g; Fiber: 1.8g

Instant Pot Cherry Compote

Serves: 8
Preparation Time: 5 minutes
Cooking Time: 15 minutes

Ingredients
- 1 package frozen cherries
- 2 tablespoon lemon juice
- ¾ cup sugar
- 2 tablespoon cornstarch
- 2 tablespoons water
- ¼ teaspoon almond extract

Instructions
1. Place the cherries, lemon juice and sugar in the Instant Pot. Stir to combine everything.
2. Close the lid and press the Manual button. Adjust the cooking time to 10 minutes.
3. Do natural pressure release.
4. Meanwhile, mix the cornstarch, water and almond extract.
5. Once the lid is open, press the Sauté button and pour the slurry over the cherries.
6. Stir and allow to simmer until the sauce thickens

Nutrition information:
Calories per serving: 46; Carbohydrates: 11.61g; Protein: 0.04g; Fat: 0.03g; Fiber: 0.1g

Steamed Keto Chocolate Cake

Serves: 12
Preparation Time: 10 minutes
Cooking Time: 30 minutes

Ingredients
- ¾ cup stevia sweetener
- 1 ½ cups all-purpose flour
- ¼ cup protein powder, chocolate or vanilla flavor
- 2/3 cup cocoa powder, unsweetened
- ¼ teaspoon baking powder
- ¼ teaspoon salt
- ½ cup unsalted butter, melted
- 4 large eggs
- ¾ cup heavy cream
- 1 teaspoon vanilla extract

Instructions
1. Place a steamer in the Instant Pot and pour a cup of water.
2. In a bowl, mix the sweetener, flour, protein powder, cocoa powder, baking powder, and salt.
3. Add the butter, eggs, cream, and vanilla extract.
4. Pour the batter into a dish that will fit inside the Instant Pot.
5. Place on the steamer and close the lid.
6. Press the Manual button and adjust the cooking time for 30 minutes.
7. Do natural pressure release.

Nutrition information:
Calories per serving: 253; Carbohydrates: 5.1g; Protein: 17.3g; Fat: 29.5g; Fiber: 2.4g

Instant Pot Raspberry Curd

Serves: 6
Preparation Time: 10 minutes
Cooking Time: 10 minutes

Ingredients
- 12 ounces raspberries
- 2 tablespoon lemon juice
- 1 cup sugar
- 2 egg yolks
- 2 tablespoons butter

Instructions
1. Place the raspberries, lemon juice and sugar in the Instant Pot.
2. Close the lid and press the Manual button.
3. Adjust the cooking time to 5 minutes.
4. Once the pressure cooker stops cooking, do natural pressure release and open the lid.
5. Strain the raspberries to puree and remove large lumps and seeds. Discard the seeds.
6. In another bowl, beat the egg yolks and add the raspberry puree. Return to the Instant Pot.
7. Without the lid on, press the Sauté button and stir constantly.
8. Add the butter and wait for the mixture to thicken.

Nutrition information:
Calories per serving: 148; Carbohydrates: 23.96g; Protein: 1.64g; Fat: 5.72g; Fiber: 3.7g

Steamed Lemon Cake

Serves: 8
Preparation Time: 10 minutes
Cooking Time: 30 minutes

Ingredients
- ½ cup all-purpose flour
- 1 ½ cups almond flour
- 3 tablespoon white sugar
- 2 teaspoon baking powder
- ½ teaspoon xanthan gum
- ½ cup whipping cream
- ½ cup butter, melted
- 1 tablespoon juice, freshly squeezed
- Zest from one large lemon
- 2 eggs

Instructions
1. Place a steamer in the Instant Pot and pour a cup of water.
2. In a bowl, mix all the ingredients until well combined.
3. Pour the batter into a dish that will fit inside the Instant Pot.
4. Put aluminum foil on top.
5. Place on the steamer and close the lid.
6. Press the Manual button and adjust the cooking time for 30 minutes.
7. Do natural pressure release.

Nutrition information:
Calories per serving: 350; Carbohydrates: 11.1g; Protein: 17.6 g; Fat: 32.6g; Fiber: 4.9g

Instant Pot Chocolate Lava Cake

Serves: 12
Preparation Time: 10 minutes
Cooking Time: 15 minutes

Ingredients
- 1 ½ cup white sugar, divided
- ½ cup all-purpose flour
- 5 tablespoon unsweetened cocoa powder
- ½ teaspoon salt
- 1 teaspoon baking powder

- 3 whole eggs
- 3 egg yolks
- ½ cup butter, melted
- 1 teaspoon vanilla extract
- 2 cups hot water
- 4 ounces sugar-free chocolate chips

Instructions
1. Place a steamer in the Instant Pot and pour a cup of water.
2. In a bowl, mix all the ingredients until well combined.
3. Pour the batter into a dish that will fit inside the Instant Pot.
4. Place on the steamer and close the lid.
5. Press the Manual button and adjust the cooking time for 15 minutes.
6. Do natural pressure release.

Nutrition information:
Calories per serving: 157; Carbohydrates: 5.5g; Protein: 10.6g; Fat: 13g; Fiber: 2.6g

Mocha Pudding Cake

Serves: 3
Preparation Time: 5 minutes
Cooking Time: 30 minutes

Ingredients
- ¾ cup butter, cut into chunks
- 2 ounces unsweetened chocolate, chopped
- ½ cup heavy cream
- 2 tablespoon instant coffee
- 1 teaspoon vanilla extract
- 1/3 cup all-purpose
- 4 tablespoon cocoa powder, unsweetened
- 1/8 teaspoon salt
- 5 large eggs
- 2/3 cup white sugar

Instructions
1. Place a steamer in the Instant Pot and pour a cup of water.
2. In a bowl, mix all the ingredients until well combined.
3. Pour the batter into a dish that will fit inside the Instant Pot.
4. Put aluminum foil on top.
5. Place on the steamer and close the lid.
6. Press the Manual button and adjust the cooking time for 30 minutes.
7. Do natural pressure release.

Nutrition information:
Calories per serving: 414; Carbohydrates: 3.8g; Protein: 10.9g; Fat: 38.9g; Fiber:0.9 g

Instant Pot Basic Steamed Vanilla Cake

Serves: 12
Preparation Time: 10 minutes
Cooking Time: 30 minutes

Ingredients
- 1 ½ cups all-purpose flour
- ¾ cup stevia sweetener
- 2/3 cup protein powder, vanilla powder
- ¼ teaspoon salt
- 2 teaspoon baking powder
- ½ cup unsalted butter, melted
- ¾ cup heavy cream
- 4 large eggs
- 1 teaspoon vanilla extract

Instructions
1. Place a steamer in the Instant Pot and pour a cup of water.
2. In a bowl, mix all the ingredients until well combined.
3. Pour the batter into a dish that will fit inside the Instant Pot.
4. Put aluminum foil on top.
5. Place on the steamer and close the lid.
6. Press the Manual button and adjust the cooking time for 30 minutes.
7. Do natural pressure release.

Nutrition information:
Calories per serving: 162; Carbohydrates: 4.1g; Protein: 11.6g; Fat: 12.3g; Fiber:0.5 g

Steamed Dark Chocolate Cake

Serves: 10
Preparation Time: 15 minutes
Cooking Time: 30 minutes

Ingredients
- 1 cup all-purpose flour
- ½ cup cocoa powder
- ½ cup white sugar
- 3 tablespoon whey protein powder, unflavored
- 1 ½ teaspoon baking powder
- ¼ teaspoon salt
- 3 large eggs
- 2/3 cup unsweetened almond milk
- 6 tablespoons butter, melted
- ¾ teaspoon vanilla extract
- 1/3 cup sugar-free chocolate chips

Instructions
1. Place a steamer in the Instant Pot and pour a cup of water.
2. In a bowl, mix all the ingredients except for the chocolate chips.
3. Pour the batter into a dish that will fit inside the Instant Pot.
4. Sprinkle with the chocolate chips on top and give a swirl.
5. Put aluminum foil on top.
6. Place on the steamer and close the lid.
7. Press the Manual button and adjust the cooking time for 30 minutes.
8. Do natural pressure release.

Nutrition information:
Calories per serving: 205; Carbohydrates:8.42 g; Protein: 7.37g; Fat: 16.79g; Fiber: 4.1g

Cinnamon Blondie Pecan Bars

Serves: 16
Preparation Time: 15 minutes
Cooking Time: 30 minutes

Ingredients
- 1 cup white sugar
- 6 tablespoon unsalted butter, melted
- 3 large eggs
- 2 teaspoon vanilla extract
- 1 ½ cups all-purpose flour

- ¼ teaspoon salt
- 1 tablespoon cinnamon
- 1 teaspoon baking powder
- 2 tablespoon unsalted butter
- ¼ cup heavy whipping cream
- 1 cup pecans, chopped

Instructions
1. Place a steamer in the Instant Pot and pour a cup of water.
2. In a bowl, whisk the sugar and butter until well combined.
3. Add the eggs and vanilla extract.
4. Stir in the flour, salt, cinnamon, baking powder, and butter.
5. Pour the batter into a dish that will fit inside the Instant Pot.
6. Put aluminum foil on top.
7. Place on the steamer and close the lid.
8. Press the Manual button and adjust the cooking time for 30 minutes.
9. Do natural pressure release.
10. Allow to cool in the fridge.
11. Garnish with whip cream and pecans on top.

Nutrition information:
Calories per serving:190.6; Carbohydrates: 1.9g; Protein: 4.42g; Fat: 20.56g; Fiber:0 g

Pumpkin Pie Pudding

Serves: 6
Preparation Time: 5 minutes
Cooking Time: 10 minutes

Ingredients
- 2 cups pumpkin, mashed
- 2 cups full-fat milk
- ¾ cup brown sugar
- ½ cup whole wheat flour
- 2 large eggs, beaten
- 2 tablespoon grass-fed butter
- 2 ½ teaspoon pumpkin pie extract
- 2 teaspoon vanilla extract

Instructions
1. Place all ingredients in the Instant Pot.
2. Give a good stir.
3. Close the lid.
4. Press the Manual button and adjust the cooking time for 10 minutes.
5. Do natural pressure release.

Nutrition information:
Calories per serving:229; Carbohydrates:33 g; Protein: 6g; Fat: 9g; Fiber: 2g

Easy Instant Pot Cheesecake

Serves: 6
Preparation Time: 10 minutes
Cooking Time: 30 minutes

Ingredients
- 3 8-ounce cream cheese, room temperature
- 1 cup white sugar
- 3 eggs
- ½ tablespoon vanilla extract

Instructions
1. Place a steamer in the Instant Pot and pour a cup of water.
2. In a bowl, mix all the ingredients until well combined.
3. Pour the batter into a springform pan that will fit inside the Instant Pot.
4. Put aluminum foil on top.
5. Place on the steamer and close the lid.
6. Press the Manual button and adjust the cooking time for 30 minutes.
7. Do natural pressure release.

Nutrition information:
Calories per serving: 264; Carbohydrates:3g; Protein: 9.1g; Fat: 15.8g; Fiber: 0g

Apple Streusel Dessert

Serves: 8
Preparation Time: 10 minutes
Cooking Time: 30 minutes

Ingredients
- 6 cups sliced, peeled, and cored tart apples
- ½ cup all-purpose flour
- ¼ teaspoon ground allspice
- 1 ¼ teaspoon ground cinnamon
- ¼ teaspoon ground nutmeg
- ¾ cup milk
- 2 tablespoons butter, softened
- ¾ cup brown sugar
- 2 large eggs, beaten
- 1 teaspoon vanilla extract
- 1/3 cup packed brown sugar
- 3 tablespoons cold butter
- ½ cup sliced almonds

Instructions
1. Place a steamer rack in the Instant Pot and pour a cup of water.
2. Place the apples in a baking dish that will fit in the Instant Pot.
3. In a mixing bowl, combine flour, allspice, cinnamon, nutmeg, milk, butter, ¾ cup brown sugar, eggs, and vanilla extract. Mix until well combined.
4. Pour over the apples and toss to coat.
5. In another bowl, combine the brown sugar, butter, and almonds.
6. Sprinkle the mixture on top of the apples.
7. Cover the baking dish with aluminum foil.
8. Close the lid and press the Steam button.
9. Adjust the cooking time to 30 minutes.
10. Do natural pressure release.

Nutrition information:
Calories per serving: 378; Carbohydrates:57 g; Protein: 5g; Fat: 16g; Fiber: 3g

Hot Fudge Sundae Cake

Serves: 12
Preparation Time: 10 minutes
Cooking Time: 30 minutes

Ingredients
- 1 ¾ cups packed brown sugar, divided
- 1 cup whole wheat flour
- 5 tablespoons baking cocoa, divided
- 2 teaspoons baking powder
- ½ teaspoon salt
- 2 tablespoons butter, melted
- ½ cup milk

- ½ teaspoon vanilla extract
- 1/8 teaspoon almond extract
- ½ cup boiling water
- 4 teaspoon instant coffee granules

Instructions
1. Place a steamer in the Instant Pot and pour a cup of water.
2. In a bowl, mix all the ingredients until well combined.
3. Pour the batter into a dish that will fit inside the Instant Pot.
4. Put aluminum foil on top.
5. Place on the steamer and close the lid.
6. Press the Manual button and adjust the cooking time for 30 minutes.
7. Do natural pressure release.

Nutrition information:
Calories per serving: 255; Carbohydrates: 48g; Protein: 3g; Fat: 7g; Fiber: 1g

Cranberry Stuffed Apples

Serves: 5
Preparation Time: 10 minutes
Cooking Time: 30 minutes

Ingredients
- 5 medium apples, cored
- 1/3 cup fresh cranberries, chopped
- 2 tablespoons walnuts, chopped
- ¼ cup packed brown sugar
- ¼ teaspoon ground cinnamon
- 1/8 teaspoon ground nutmeg

Instructions
1. Place a steamer basket in the Instant Pot and pour a cup of water.
2. Place the cored apples in a baking dish that will fit in the Instant Pot.
3. In a mixing bowl, combine the cranberries, walnuts, sugar, cinnamon, and nutmeg.
4. Spoon the mixture into the hollowed center of the apples.
5. Place an aluminum foil on top of the baking dish.
6. Place on the steamer rack.
7. Close the lid and press the Steam button.
8. Adjust the cooking time to 30 minutes.
9. Do natural pressure release.

Nutrition information:
Calories per serving: 136; Carbohydrates: 31g; Protein: 1g; Fat: 2g; Fiber: 4g

Gingerbread Pudding Cake

Serves: 8
Preparation Time: 15 minutes
Cooking Time: 30 minutes

Ingredients
- 1 cup water
- ½ cup molasses
- ¼ cup butter, softened
- ¼ cup granulated sugar
- 1 large egg white
- 1 teaspoon vanilla extract
- 1 ¼ cups whole wheat flour
- ¾ teaspoon baking soda
- ¼ teaspoon salt
- ½ teaspoon ground ginger
- ½ teaspoon ground cinnamon
- 1/8 teaspoon ground nutmeg
- ¼ teaspoon ground allspice
- ½ cup chopped pecans

Instructions
1. Place a steamer in the Instant Pot and pour a cup of water.
2. Combine water and molasses in a mixing bowl. Stir in the softened butter, granulated sugar, egg white, and vanilla. Mix until fluffy.
3. In another bowl, combine the flour, baking soda, and salt. Add the ginger, cinnamon, nutmeg, and allspice.
4. Mix the wet ingredients to the dry ingredients until well combined.
5. Fold in the pecans.
6. Pour into a baking dish that will fit inside the Instant Pot and sprinkle with top brown sugar.
7. Put aluminum foil on top of the baking dish.
8. Place on the steamer rack and press the Steam button.
9. Adjust the cooking time to 30 minutes.
10. Do natural pressure release.
11. Allow to cool before slicing.

Nutrition information:
Calories per serving:431; Carbohydrates: 48g; Protein: 3g; Fat: 25g; Fiber:1 g

Slow Cooker Berry Cobbler

Serves: 8
Preparation Time: 10 minutes
Cooking Time: 30 minutes

Ingredients
- 1 ¼ cups whole wheat flour, divided
- 1 cup and 2 tablespoons sugar, divided
- ¼ teaspoon ground cinnamon
- 1 teaspoon baking powder
- 1 large eggs
- 2 tablespoons canola oil
- ¼ cups fat-free milk
- 1/8 teaspoon salt
- 2 cups fresh raspberries
- 2 cups fresh blueberries

Instructions
1. Place a steamer in the Instant Pot and pour a cup of water.
2. In a mixing bowl, combine 1 cup of flour, 2 tablespoons of sugar, cinnamon, and baking powder.
3. In another bowl, mix the egg, oil, and milk.
4. Add the wet ingredients to the dry ingredients and stir constantly until well combined.
5. Pour the batter into a dish that will fit inside the Instant Pot.
6. In another bowl, toss together with salt and the berries.
7. Spread berries on top of the batter.
8. Place aluminum foil on top of the baking dish.
9. Place on the steamer rack.
10. Close the lid and cook on press the Steam button.
11. Adjust the cooking time to 30 minutes.
12. Do natural pressure release.

Nutrition information:

Calories per serving:260; Carbohydrates:53 g; Protein: 4g; Fat: 5g; Fiber: 3g

Pink Grapefruit Cheesecake

Serves: 6
Preparation Time: 10 minutes
Cooking Time: 30 minutes
Ingredients
- ¾ cup graham cracker crumbs
- 1 tablespoon + 2/3 cup sugar, divided
- 1 teaspoon grated grapefruit peel
- ¼ teaspoon ground ginger
- 2 ½ tablespoons butter, melted
- 2 packages cream cheese, softened
- ½ cup sour cream
- 2 tablespoons pink grapefruit juice
- 2 large eggs, beaten

Instructions
1. Place a steamer basket in the Instant Pot and pour a cup of water.
2. Wrap a springform pan with foil to prevent the cheesecake from leaking from the pan. Make sure that the pan will fit inside the Instant Pot.
3. In a bowl, mix the graham cracker crumbs, 1 tablespoon sugar, grapefruit peel, ginger, and butter. Mix until well combined. Press the crust mixture into the base of the springform pan. Set aside to cool inside the fridge.
4. In another bowl, beat the remaining sugar and cream cheese. Add the sour cream, grapefruit juice, and eggs. Whisk until well combined.
5. Pour the cheesecake mixture into the springform pan.
6. Place on top of the steamer rack and close the lid.
7. Press the Steam button and adjust the cooking time to 30 minutes.
8. Do natural pressure release.

Nutrition information:
Calories per serving: 515; Carbohydrates: 39g; Protein: 8g; Fat: 37g; Fiber: 0g

Maple Crème Brulee

Serves: 3
Preparation Time: 10 minutes
Cooking Time: 30 minutes
Ingredients
- 3 large egg yolks, beaten
- ½ cup packed brown sugar
- ¼ teaspoon ground cinnamon
- 1 1/3 cups heavy whipping cream, warm
- ½ teaspoon maple flavoring
- 1 ½ teaspoon sugar for topping

Instructions
1. Place a steamer in the Instant Pot and pour a cup of boiling water.
2. In a bowl, whisk the yolks, sugar, and cinnamon. Stir in the warm cream to the yolk mixture.
3. Stir in the maple flavoring.
4. Ladle the mixture into ramekins and sprinkle sugar for the topping.
5. Place the ramekins in the steamer basket.
6. Close the lid and press the Steam button.
7. Adjust the cooking time to 30 minutes.
8. Do natural pressure release.
9. Remove the ramekins and allow to cool in the fridge for 10 minutes.

Nutrition information:
Calories per serving: 578; Carbohydrates: 44g; Protein: 5g; Fat: 44g; Fiber: 0g

Sweet Rice Pudding

Serves: 4
Preparation Time: 10 minutes
Cooking Time: 15 minutes
Ingredients
- 1 ¼ cups milk
- ½ cup uncooked rice
- ½ cups brown sugar
- ½ cup raisin
- 1 teaspoon ground cinnamon
- 1 teaspoon butter, melted
- 2 eggs, beaten
- 1 teaspoon vanilla extract
- ¾ teaspoon lemon extract
- 1 cup heavy whipping cream

Instructions
1. Place all ingredients except the whipping cream in the Instant Pot.
2. Give a good stir to incorporate all ingredients.
3. Close the lid and press the Manual button.
4. Adjust the cooking time to 15 minutes
5. Allow to chill in the fridge before serving.
6. Serve with whipping cream

Nutrition information:
Calories per serving:437; Carbohydrates: 63g; Protein: 8g; Fat:17 g; Fiber: 1g

Coconut, Cranberry, And Quinoa Crockpot Breakfast

Serves: 4
Preparation Time: 5 minutes
Cooking Time: 20 minutes
Ingredients
- 2 ½ cups coconut water
- ¼ cup slivered almonds
- ½ cup coconut meat
- 1 cup quinoa, rinsed
- ½ cup dried cranberries
- 1 tablespoon vanilla
- ¼ cup honey

Instructions
1. Place all ingredients except the whipping cream in the Instant Pot.
2. Give a good stir to incorporate all ingredients.
3. Close the lid and press the Manual button.
4. Adjust the cooking time to 20 minutes
5. Allow to chill in the fridge before serving.

Nutrition information:
Calories per serving: 478; Carbohydrates:66.1 g; Protein: 6.4g; Fat:25.8 g; Fiber: 8.1g

Caramel and Pear Pudding

Serves: 7
Preparation Time: 10 minutes
Cooking Time: 15 minutes
Ingredients

- ½ cup sugar
- ½ teaspoon ground cinnamon
- 1 ½ teaspoons baking powder
- 1/8 teaspoon ground cloves
- ¼ teaspoon salt
- 3/4 cup milk
- 4 medium pears, peeled and cubed
- ½ cup pecans, chopped
- ¾ cup brown sugar
- ¼ cup softened butter

Instructions
1. Place all ingredients in the Instant Pot.
2. Give a good stir to incorporate all ingredients.
3. Close the lid and press the Manual button.
4. Adjust the cooking time to 15 minutes
5. Allow to chill in the fridge before serving.

Nutrition information:
Calories per serving:274; Carbohydrates:47 g; Protein: 3g; Fat: 9g; Fiber: 3g

Double Dark Chocolate Cake

Serves: 6
Preparation Time: 10 minutes
Cooking Time: 25 minutes

Ingredients
- 4 drops liquid stevia
- 2 tablespoon raw cacao nibs
- ¼ cups unsweetened applesauce
- 2 tablespoon almond milk, unsweetened
- ½ cup coconut milk, full fat
- 1 large egg
- ½ teaspoon vanilla
- ½ cup cacao powder
- ½ cup raw honey
- 2 tablespoon tapioca flour
- 1 cup almond flour

Instructions
1. Place a steamer basket in the Instant Pot.
2. In a mixing bowl, combine all ingredients.
3. Pour into a baking dish that will fit in the Instant Pot.
4. Place aluminum foil on top.
5. Place on top of the steamer basket.
6. Close the lid and press the Steam button.
7. Adjust the cooking time to 30 minutes.
8. Do natural pressure release.

Nutrition information:
Calories per serving: 267; Carbohydrates: 15.6g; Protein: 18.1g; Fat: 46.6g; Fiber: 72.1g

Apple Cinnamon Cake

Serves: 6
Preparation Time: 10 minutes
Cooking Time: 30 minutes

Ingredients
- 1 teaspoon fresh nutmeg, grated
- 1 tablespoon vanilla
- 1 medium peeled apple, cored and diced
- 1 large egg
- ½ cup raw honey
- ¼ cup coconut oil, melted
- 1 teaspoon cinnamon
- ¼ cup arrowroot powder
- ½ teaspoon baking soda
- ½ teaspoon salt
- 2 cups almond flour

Instructions
1. Place a steamer basket in the Instant Pot.
2. In a mixing bowl, combine all ingredients.
3. Pour into a baking dish that will fit in the Instant Pot.
4. Place aluminum foil on top.
5. Place on top of the steamer basket.
6. Close the lid and press the Steam button.
7. Adjust the cooking time to 30 minutes.
8. Do natural pressure release.

Nutrition information:
Calories per serving:204; Carbohydrates: 29.1g; Protein: 0.9g; Fat: 10.4g; Fiber: 1.2g

Fruit Salad Jam

Serves: 6
Preparation Time: 5 minutes
Cooking Time: 15 minutes

Ingredients
- ½ teaspoon cinnamon
- 1 medium apple, diced
- 1 medium oranges, peeled
- 1 cup blueberries
- 1 cup sugar
- Zest of ½ lemon
- 1 ½ cups water

Instructions
1. Place all ingredients in the Instant Pot.
2. Give a good stir.
3. Close the lid and press the Manual button.
4. Adjust the cooking time to 10 minutes.
5. Do natural pressure release.
6. Once the lid is open, press the Sauté button and simmer to reduce the sauce.

Nutrition information:
Calories per serving: 131; Carbohydrates: 33.6g; Protein: 0.7g; Fat: 0.2g; Fiber: 2.1g

Pumpkin Spice Chocolate Chip Cookies

Serves: 6
Preparation Time: 10 minutes
Cooking Time: 30 minutes

Ingredients
- ½ cup chocolate chips, semi-sweet
- 1 tablespoon pumpkin pie spice
- 1 teaspoon baking soda
- 2 teaspoons vanilla
- ¼ cup coconut oil
- ¼ cup raw honey
- 3 tablespoon almond butter
- ½ cup pumpkin puree
- 1 ½ cup all-purpose flour

Instructions
1. Place a steamer basket in the Instant Pot.
2. In a mixing bowl, combine all ingredients.
3. Pour into a baking dish that will fit in the Instant Pot.
4. Place aluminum foil on top.
5. Place on top of the steamer basket.
6. Close the lid and press the Steam button.

7. Adjust the cooking time to 30 minutes.
8. Do natural pressure release.
Nutrition information:
Calories per serving: 489; Carbohydrates: 58.9g; Protein: 9.4g; Fat: 25.5g; Fiber: 3.2g

Instant Pot Sweetened Rhubarb

Serves: 6
Preparation Time: 5 minutes
Cooking Time: 15 minutes
Ingredients
- ½ cups strawberries, fresh and cleaned
- 2 medium lemon, juiced
- 1 teaspoon vanilla
- 1 medium orange, juiced
- 1 ½ pounds rhubarb, sliced into segments
- 1 cup water
- 2 cups raw honey

Instructions
1. Place all ingredients in the Instant Pot.
2. Give a good stir.
3. Close the lid and press the Manual button.
4. Adjust the cooking time to 10 minutes.
5. Do natural pressure release.
6. Once the lid is open, press the Sauté button and simmer to reduce the sauce.

Nutrition information:
Calories per serving: 484; Carbohydrates: 130g; Protein: 0.9g; Fat: 0.3g; Fiber: 2.8g

Appendix : Recipes Index

10-Minute Mushroom Broth 69
   13-Bean Soup 33
   15-Bean Soup 33
   15-Bean Tailgate Chili in Instant Pot 34
   3-Ingredient Bone Broth 70
   3-Ingredient Pork Chops 105
   40-Clove Chicken 57
   5-Ingredient Cheesy Egg Bake 13
   5-Ingredient Shakshuka 27

A

African Peanut Butter Beef Stew 78
Apple Cinnamon Cake 125
Apple Delicata Squash Porridge 18
Apple Streusel Dessert 122
Aromatic Rosemary Garlic Potatoes 113
Asian Chicken Stock 63
Asian Coconut Rice Pudding 117
Asian Fish and Vegetables 83
Asian Garlic and Honey Chicken 58
Asian Pot Roast 90
Asian Scrambled Eggs 23
Asian Sesame Noodles 115
Asian Short Ribs 94
Asian Soup Stock 65
Asparagus and Chive Frittata 24

B

Bacon and Broccoli Quiche 24
Bacon and Cheese Crustless Quiche 11
Bacon Ranch Potatoes 10
Baked Eggs with Chorizo 29
Baked with Beans with Bacon 41
Balsamic Orange Chicken Drumsticks 61
Balsamic Pot Roast 91
Balsamic Spiced Apple Pork 107
Banana French Toast 17
Banana Walnut Steel-Cut Oats 52
Basic Beef Stock 63
Basic Braised Beef Short Ribs 94
Basic Instant Pot Egg Salad Recipe 21
Basic Instant Pot Millet 51
Basic Instant Pot Quinoa 49
Basic Instant Pot Risotto 46
Basic Vegetable Stock 63
BBQ Beef Ribs 93
BBQ Pulled Pork 102
Beans and Squash Minestrone 41
Beans and Tomato Stew 78
Beans with Cajun Sausages Soup 36
Beef Barley Soup 48
Beef Barley Stew with Sour Cream 97
Beef Borscht Soup 72
Beefy Instant Pot Congee 48
Beer-Braised Pulled Ham 104
Belizean Stewed Chicken 58
Black Bean Soup with Poblano Chilies 38
Black Eyed Peas and Ham 32
Blueberry Breakfast Oats 19
Blueberry French Toast 20
Brazilian Beef Stew (Feijoada) 97
Breakfast Espresso Oatmeal 13
Breakfast Green Chile 16
Brothy Beans with Cream 37
Brown Rice Congee with Shiitake Mushrooms 49
Browned Chicken Broth 70
Brussels Sprouts With Pine Nuts and Pomegranate Seeds 114
Buffalo Pork Chops 103
Butter Bean Ragout 38
Butter Chicken Murgh Makhani 53
Butternut and Cauliflower Stew 75
Butternut Squash Risotto 47

C

Cannellini and Tomato Soup 39
Cannellini Beans Stew with Chicken and Dried Cherries 39
Cannellini Beans with Shrimp and Tomatoes 37
Caramel and Pear Pudding 124
Cheesy Chili Mac 81
Cheesy Egg Bake 11
Cheesy Egg Casserole 25
Chicken and Rice 43
Chicken and Sweet Potato Chipotle Soup 73
Chicken Barley Soup 48
Chicken Faux Pho 74
Chicken Feet Stock 68
Chicken with Mushrooms and Mustard 60
Chicken with White Wine Mushroom Sauce 59
Chile Pork Stew 106
Chili Lime Chicken 56
Chili Verde Recipe 104
Chinese BBQ Pork (Char Siu) 107
Chinese Master Stock 69
Chinese Pork Stock 66
Chinese-Style Steamed Ginger Scallion Fish 85
Chives and Eggs Casserole 28
Chorizo, Kale and Apple Frittata 31
Chunky and Beanless Beef Chili 92
Cilantro Lime Rice 43
Cinnamon Blondie Pecan Bars 121
Clams and Corn 87
Classic Beef Bone Broth 71
Classic Beef Chili 80
Classic Chicken Bone Broth 70
Classic Pork Broth 66
Classic Pot Roast 91
Coconut Curry Sea Bass 89
Coconut Pina Colada Pudding 119
Coconut, Cranberry, And Quinoa Crockpot Breakfast 124
Coffee Pork Ribs 100
Corned Beef Brisket 99
Crabs in Coconut Milk 86
Cranberry Maple Orange Pork Chops 104
Cranberry Stuffed Apples 123
Creamy Artichoke, Garlic, And Zucchini 110
Creamy Bean and Artichoke Dip 115

Creamy Cheese Au Gratin 113
Creamy Haddock with Kale 89
Creamy Millet Breakfast Porridge 51
Creamy Thai Coconut Chicken Soup 76
Crockpot Pumpkin Chili 109
Crockpot Summer Veggies Side Dish 110
Crustless And Meaty Quiche 18
Cuban Black Bean Soup 72
Curried Squash Stew 108

D

Double Dark Chocolate Cake 125
Dulce De Leche 118

E

Easy Beef and Broccoli Stir Fry 97
Easy Corn Chowder 78
Easy Instant Pot Cheesecake 122
Easy Instant Pot Poached Eggs 25
Easy Irish Oatmeal 12
Easy Lazy Pressure Cooker Chili 34
Easy Savory Turkey Stock 71
Easy Venison Broth 66
Egg and Broccoli Casserole 20
Egg Masala Curry 30
Eggs and Chorizo 23
Eggs Benedict Casserole 11
Eggs En Cocotte 13
Eggs in Pots with Smoked Salmon Casserole 30
Enchilada Chicken Stew 79
Ethiopian Spinach and Lentil Soup 74
Extra Thick Almond Milk Yogurt 19

F

Fall-Of-The-Bones Ribs 101
Farro And Cherry Salad 111
Fast Pressure Cooker Hazelnut Flan 118
Festive Chicken Ginger Congee 49
Fish Coconut Curry 84
Fish with Orange and Ginger Sauce 84
Five Spice Beef Stew 96
French Baked Eggs 14
French Style Chicken Potatoes 62
French Toast Casserole 16
Fruit Salad Jam 125
Fruited Steel-Cut Breakfast Oats 13

G

Garden Harvest Soup 72
Gigante Beans in Tomato Sauce 40
Ginger Pork Shogayaki 106
Gingerbread Pudding Cake 123
Grains and Kale Salad 112
Greek Gigante Beans 33
Greek Pork Ribs 101
Greek Style Beef Stew 91
Green Chili Mahi Mahi 84

H

Ham and Cheese Casserole 14
Ham, Egg, And Cheese Casserole 18
Hearty and Creamy Broccoli Soup 75
Herbed Crustless Quiche 23
Hibachi Fried Rice 44
Honey Bourbon Chicken 53
Honey Lime Ginger Pork Chops 103
Honey Sesame Chicken 54
Honey Teriyaki Chicken 57
Hoshi Shiitake Dashi 64
Hot Fudge Sundae Cake 122
Hungarian Pork Paprikash 106

I

Indian Coconut Kale Curry 109
Indian Green Beans and Potatoes 36
Indian Scrambled Eggs 22
Indian Vegetable Rice 43
Instant Pot "Baked" Apples 116
Instant Pot Alfredo Chicken Noodles 60
Instant Pot Apple Spice Oats 52
Instant Pot Asian Pork Belly 105
Instant Pot Asparagus Risotto 46
Instant Pot Bacon and Broccoli Frittata 26
Instant Pot Banana Bread 20
Instant Pot Barbecue Ribs 101
Instant Pot Basic Congee (Jook) 49
Instant Pot Basic Steamed Vanilla Cake 121
Instant Pot Basic Steamed Vegetables 110
Instant Pot BBQ Chicken with Potatoes 57
Instant Pot Beef Burgundy 94
Instant Pot Beef Mechado 91
Instant Pot Beef Ragu 98
Instant Pot Boiled Octopus 88
Instant Pot Bread Pudding 17
Instant Pot Breakfast Coconut Yogurt 18
Instant Pot Breakfast Frittatas 21
Instant Pot Buckwheat Porridge 49
Instant Pot Cajun Chicken and Rice 44
Instant Pot Cajun Peanuts 109
Instant Pot Carne Guisada 79
Instant Pot Carne Guisada 96
Instant Pot Cashew Chicken 57
Instant Pot Cauliflower Curry 108
Instant Pot Cauliflower Soup 108
Instant Pot Cheddar, Broccoli, And Potato Soup 73
Instant Pot Cheese Steak 92
Instant Pot Cheeseburger Soup 75
Instant Pot Cherry Compote 120
Instant Pot Chicken Adobo 55
Instant Pot Chicken Biryani 56
Instant Pot Chicken Cacciatore 53
Instant Pot Chicken Creole 59
Instant Pot Chicken Piccata 60
Instant Pot Chicken Tortilla Soup 73
Instant Pot Chipotle Chili 80
Instant Pot Chocolate Lava Cake 120
Instant Pot Coconut Oatmeal 52
Instant Pot Coddled Eggs 29
Instant Pot Cowboy Chili 80
Instant Pot Crack Chicken 55
Instant Pot Cranberry Sauce 68
Instant Pot Creamy Mushroom Wild Rice Soup 45
Instant Pot Crème Brule 117
Instant Pot Cuban Black Beans 36

Instant Pot Curried Pork Chops 103
Instant Pot Deviled Eggs 25
Instant Pot Drunken Beans 35
Instant Pot Easy Baked Beans 32
Instant Pot Easy Mushroom Chili 109
Instant Pot Easy Scallops 88
Instant Pot Egg Cups 21
Instant Pot Egg Custard 22
Instant Pot Egg Muffins 21
Instant Pot Eggs in Marinara Sauce 22
Instant Pot Football Chili 72
Instant Pot French Onion Soup 110
Instant Pot Goat Stew 76
Instant Pot Goulash 79
Instant Pot Green Chili Stew 80
Instant Pot Green Split Pea Soup 34
Instant Pot Ground Beef Shawarma Rice 44
Instant Pot Ham and Bean Soup 35
Instant Pot Ham and Potato Soup 77
Instant Pot Ham Bone Broth 69
Instant Pot Hard Boiled Egg Loaf 26
Instant Pot Hard Boiled Eggs 18
Instant Pot Herb Stock 66
Instant Pot Herbed Chicken 61
Instant Pot Hong Kong Egg Custard 25
Instant Pot Huevos Rancheros 12
Instant Pot Hummus 35
Instant Pot Jamaican Jerk Chicken 59
Instant Pot Jambalaya 86
Instant Pot Kalua Pig 101
Instant Pot Kimchi Stew (Korean Kimchi Jjigae) 77
Instant Pot Korean Glazed Ribs 100
Instant Pot Lasagna Soup 74
Instant Pot Lemon Orzo Soup 26
Instant Pot Lobster Roll 88
Instant Pot Mediterranean Fish 83
Instant Pot Mexican Rice 45
Instant Pot Millet Porridge 51
Instant Pot Mok Pa 85
Instant Pot Mongolian Beef 97
Instant Pot Mongolian Chicken 54
Instant Pot Mushroom Broth 68
Instant Pot Mushroom Risotto 45
Instant Pot Mussels 88
Instant Pot Nikujaga 96
Instant Pot Orange Chicken 58
Instant Pot Oreo Cheesecake 116
Instant Pot Paleo Carnitas 102
Instant Pot Pearl Barley 47
Instant Pot Perfectly Soft-Boiled Eggs 21
Instant Pot Pineapple Ham 104
Instant Pot Poached Salmon 82
Instant Pot Poblano Cheese Frittata 23
Instant Pot Porcini Risotto 46
Instant Pot Pork Adobo 103
Instant Pot Pork Stroganoff 105
Instant Pot Pork Vindaloo 76
Instant Pot Quinoa Pilaf 50
Instant Pot Raspberry Curd 120

Instant Pot Red Beans and Rice 35
Instant Pot Refried Beans 33
Instant Pot Ribs 100
Instant Pot Rice 43
Instant Pot Rice Pilaf 44
Instant Pot Rotisserie Chicken 54
Instant Pot Salmon Fillet 83
Instant Pot Sauerbraten (German-Style Beef) 92
Instant Pot Scotch Broth 64
Instant Pot Scrambled Eggs 22
Instant Pot Seafood Stew 87
Instant Pot Shellfish Stock 68
Instant Pot Shredded Chicken 54
Instant Pot Shrimp Boil 86
Instant Pot Shrimps 86
Instant Pot Sloppy Joes 98
Instant Pot Slow Cooker Chocolate Oatmeal 13
Instant Pot Southwest Biscuit Egg Bake 25
Instant Pot Spanish Rice 43
Instant Pot Steamed Artichoke 115
Instant Pot Strawberry Applesauce 68
Instant Pot Sweetened Rhubarb 126
Instant Pot Tuna Casserole 89
Instant Pot Turkey Chili 79
Instant Pot Turkey Chili 81
Instant Pot Vegan Stroganoff 108
Instant Pot White Stock 64
Instant Pot Zucchini Casserole 110
Instant Pot Zuppa Toscana 75
Irish Beef Stew 94
Italian Bean Stew 42
Italian Chicken Marsala 53
Italian Pot Roast 90
Italian Sausage Stew 78
Italian Short Ribs 93
Italian Tomato Meatballs 98

J

Jamaican Cornmeal Porridge 16
Japanese Dashi Stock 64
Japanese Seafood Curry 87

K

Korean Basil Beef Bowls 98
Korean Short Ribs 93
Korean Style Galbijjm 95
Korean-Style Dashi Stock 67

L

Lazy Man's Baked Beans 33
Lazy Sweet and Sour Chicken 59
Leftover Turkey Carcass Soup 70
Lemon and Dill Fish Packets 85
Lemon Blueberry Breakfast Cake 11
Lemon Mustard Chicken with Potatoes 55
Lemon Olive Chicken 53
Lemon Shrimps with Veggies and Parmesan 89
Lemongrass and Coconut Chicken 55
Loaded Breakfast Potatoes 10
Lobster with Wine and Tomatoes 88

M

Magic Mineral Broth 67

Maple Crème Brulee 124
Maple Spice Rubbed Ribs 100
Mediterranean-Style Cod 89
Mexican Beans with Beef Soup 40
Mexican Egg Casserole 15
Mexican Eggs with Potato Hash 31
Mexican Meatball Soup 75
Mexican Quinoa with Cilantro Sauce 50
Mexican Short Ribs 95
Mexican-Style Quiche 12
Mississippi Coke Beef 92
Mixed Beans Salad 38
Mocha Pudding Cake 121
Mocha-Rubbed Roast 93
Mojo Chicken Tacos 58
Mole Beef Stew 96
Moo Shu Pork 105
Moringa Chicken Soup 55
Mushroom Gravy Sauce 65

N

Navy Bean Escarole Stew 37

O

Old Bay Fish Tacos 84
One-Minute Quinoa and Veggies 50
One-Pan Eggs and Peppers 29
Orange-Glazed Pork Chops 102

P

Pasta Cannellini with Escarole 40
Peaches and Cream Oatmeal 52
Pearl Barley Soup 48
Peppercorn Pork Brisket 106
Pepperoni and Potato Frittata 28
Pink Grapefruit Cheesecake 124
Pinto Beans with Chorizo 32
Poached Eggs in Bell Pepper Cups 15
Poor Man's Pot Roast 93
Pork Chops with Honey Mustard 103
Pork Ribs with Memphis Rub 102
Potato Bacon Egg Breakfast 27
Potato Egg Frittata 19
Pressure Cooker Mashed Potatoes 113
Proofing Whole Wheat Bread in Instant Pot 51
Puchero A La Valencia (Spanish Stew) 77
Pumpkin and Chocolate Bundt Cake 119
Pumpkin and Rice Pudding 117
Pumpkin Lentil Soup 34
Pumpkin Pie Pudding 122
Pumpkin Spice Chocolate Chip Cookies 125
Pumpkin Spice Oat Meal 52

Q

Quick Hoisin Chicken 61
Quinoa Fried Rice 50
Quinoa with Mushrooms and Vegetables 51

R

Red Lentil Chili 76
Rice Pilaf with Vegetables 112
Rice with Chicken and Broccoli 45
Risotto with Bacon and Peas 46
Roasted Cauliflower Barley Risotto 47
Roasted Chicken Stock 67

Romesco Eggs with Sausages 30
Root Beer Chicken Wings 60

S

Salmon and Rice Pilaf 82
Salmon and Veggies 82
Salmon with Lemon Caper Chimichurri 83
Saucy Spanish Chorizo and Potato Hash 10
Sausage and Egg Breakfast Casserole Burritos 15
Sausage Greens and Bean Pasta 37
Sausage, Ham, And Cheese Quiche 24
Sausages and Eggs 27
Savory Mashed Sweet Potatoes 111
Seafood Soup Stock 66
Shortcut Pork Posole 105
Shrimps in Lobsters Sauce 86
Silver Beet and Dukkah Baked Eggs 28
Simple Boiled Kidney Beans 32
Simple Boiled Pinto Beans 32
Simple Bone Broth 63
Simple Bone-In Ribs 94
Simple Breakfast Oatmeal with Brown Sugar 14
Simple Egg Casserole 27
Simple Eggplant Spread 114
Simple General Tso's Pork 106
Simple Green Beans Salad 113
Simple Instant Pot Roast 90
Simple Instant Pot Salmon 83
Simple Pressure Cooker Chickpea Hummus 114
Simple Rice Salad 115
Simple Savory Tomatoes and Eggs 31
Simple Spiced Black Beans 32
Slow Cooker Berry Cobbler 123
Smoked Pull Pork 102
Smoked Turkey Stock 64
Smokey Honey Cilantro Chicken 56
Smoking Hot Pickled Green Chilies 114
Smoky BBQ Instant Pot Ribs 100
Smothered Pork Chops 104
Sous Vide Egg Bites 21
Spice Bean and Chicken Chorizo Chili 38
Spicy Bean Soup with Sausages 40
Spicy Beans with Wilted Greens 39
Spicy Brown Rice Salad with Black Beans 116
Spicy Fava Bean Soup 41
Spicy Lemon Halibut 82
Spicy Thai Quinoa Salad 112
Spinach and Goat Cheese Risotto 47
Spinach and Ham Frittata 12
Spinach Baked Eggs with Parmesan on Toast 29
Steamed Carrot Pudding Cake 119
Steamed Crab Legs 87
Steamed Cranberry Pudding 117
Steamed Dark Chocolate Cake 121
Steamed Fish Patra Ni Maachi 90
Steamed Keto Chocolate Cake 120
Steamed Key Lime Pie 118

Steamed Lemon Cake 120
Steamed Savory Artichokes 115
Steamed Scotch Eggs 17
Steamed Shrimps and Asparagus in Instant Pot 87
Steamed Vegetables Side Dish 111
Stewed Spicy Cannellini Beans 42
Sticky Chicken and Chilies 61
Sticky Glazed Spare Ribs 100
Sunday Pot Roast 91
Sun-Dried Tomato Polenta 112
Sweet and Savory Baked Beans 36
Sweet and Smoky Short Ribs 95
Sweet and Sour Riblets 101
Sweet and Spicy Mahi Mahi 85
Sweet Apple Pudding 116
Sweet Chili Sauce Braised Pork 107
Sweet Coconut Tapioca 118
Sweet Potato Hash 10
Sweet Rice Pudding 124
Sweet Sticky Carrots 113
Swiss Chard Stem Soup 73

T

Texas Beef Chili 81
Tex-Mex Pinto Beans 35
Thai Chicken Stew 56
Thai Coconut Fish 84
Thai Soup Stock 65
Toad-in-the-hole Eggs and Tomatoes 30
Tomato and Basil Soup 108
Trail Mix Breakfast Oatmeal 14
Turkey Egg Breakfast Casserole 26
Turkey Giblet Stock 63
Turkey Soup Stock 65

V

Vanilla Apple Cinnamon Breakfast Quinoa 16
Vegan and Gluten-Free Stock 64
Vegan Beef Stock 69
Vegan Chicken Stock 69
Vegan Miso Risotto 111
Vegan Pulled "Pork" 109
Vegan Pumpkin Coffee Cake Oatmeal 19
Vegan Pumpkin Stew 108
Vegetable Beef Stew 95
Veggie Cheese Soup 109
Vietnamese Beef Bo Kho 95
Vietnamese Chicken Congee (Chao Ga) 48
Vietnamese Pho Stock 67

W

Western Omelet Quiche 14
Western Shoulder Ribs 101
White Beans and Broccoli 41
White Chicken Chili 81
Whole Food Minestrone Soup 72
Wild Alaskan Cod 84

Y

Yakitori Chicken Wings 61
Yogurt with Fruits 16

Z

Zucchini and Eggs 28

CPSIA information can be obtained
at www.ICGtesting.com
Printed in the USA
LVHW011655200221
679511LV00003B/273

9 781801 243261